MOSBY'S Workbook for the

Home Care Aide

Joan Birchenall, RN, MEd
Trenton, New Jersey

2nd Edition

Eileen Streight, RN, BSN
Hamilton, New Jersey

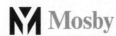 Mosby

St. Louis Philadelphia London Sydney Toronto

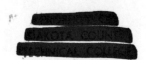

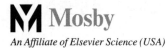

Mosby

An Affiliate of Elsevier Science (USA)

11830 Westline Industrial Drive
St. Louis, Missouri 63146

Mosby's Workbook for the Home Care Aide
SECOND EDITION

Printed in the United States of America.

International Standard Book Number 0-323-01657-X

Vice President and Publishing Director, Nursing: Sally Schrefer
Executive Editor: Susan R. Epstein
Senior Developmental Editor: Maria Broeker
Publishing Services Manager: Gayle May
Project Manager: Stephanie M. Hebenstreit
Designer: Kathi Gosche

02   03   04   05   06   KI/MV   9   8   7   6   5   4   3   2   1

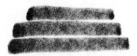

Reviewers

Evelyn Hawrylak, RN, CSW, MPA
Liaison Nurse
Mercer Street Friends Visiting Nurse Agency
Trenton, New Jersey

Cynthia McNairn, RN, BA, BScN
Professor
George Brown College
Toronto, Ontario, Canada

Illustration Credits

To the Student

How to Use This Workbook

This workbook is designed to help you gain the knowledge and skills needed to begin your career as a home care aide. All of the answers can be found in the corresponding chapters of *Mosby's Textbook for the Home Care Aide*, second edition. Each set of exercises will help you meet the chapter objectives stated in the text.

Suggestions for using the workbook successfully include:
· Read and follow directions
· Complete each assignment
· Ask your teacher for help if you have any questions or need assistance
· Use the textbook to look up answers that you don't know
· Check your answers with the correct answers provided in this workbook

This workbook gives you the opportunity to be involved in the learning process and to test yourself to see what you have learned and what you still need to study.

Contents

Questions

PART 1   **ORIENTATION TO HOME CARE**

Chapter 1	Learning About Home Care	1
Chapter 2	The Home Care Industry	4
Chapter 3	Developing Effective Communication Skills	7
Chapter 4	Understanding Your Client's Needs	12
Chapter 5	Understanding How the Body Works	15
Chapter 6	Observing, Reporting, and Recording	20
Chapter 7	Working With the Ill and Disabled	27

PART 2   **MANAGING THE HOME ENVIRONMENT**

Chapter 8	Maintaining a Safe Environment	31
Chapter 9	Maintaining a Healthy Environment	35
Chapter 10	Meeting the Client's Nutritional Needs	37

PART 3   **HOME CARE PROCEDURES**

Chapter 11	Preventing Infection/Medical Asepsis	42
Chapter 12	Body Mechanics	46
Chapter 13	Bedmaking	52
Chapter 14	Personal Care	54
Chapter 15	Elimination	61
Chapter 16	Collecting Specimens	67
Chapter 17	Measuring Vital Signs	73
Chapter 18	Special Procedures	79

PART 4   **MEETING THE CLIENT'S SPECIAL NEEDS**

Chapter 19	Caring for Older Adults	87
Chapter 20	Caring for Mothers, Infants, and Children	91
Chapter 21	Caring for Clients With Mental Illness	94
Chapter 22	Caring for Clients With Illnesses Requiring Home Care	99
Chapter 23	Caring for the Dying Client	106
Chapter 24	Emergencies	108

PART 5   **PROFESSIONAL SKILLS**

Chapter 25	Getting a Job and Keeping It	111

v

Answers

PART 1   ORIENTATION TO HOME CARE

Chapter 1	Learning About Home Care	119
Chapter 2	The Home Care Industry	120
Chapter 3	Developing Effective Communication Skills	122
Chapter 4	Understanding Your Client's Needs	124
Chapter 5	Understanding How the Body Works	127
Chapter 6	Observing, Reporting, and Recording	129
Chapter 7	Working With the Ill and Disabled	135

PART 2   MANAGING THE HOME ENVIRONMENT

Chapter 8	Maintaining a Safe Environment	136
Chapter 9	Maintaining a Healthy Environment	139
Chapter 10	Meeting the Client's Nutritional Needs	140

PART 3   HOME CARE PROCEDURES

Chapter 11	Preventing Infection/Medical Asepsis	144
Chapter 12	Body Mechanics	146
Chapter 13	Bedmaking	148
Chapter 14	Personal Care	149
Chapter 15	Elimination	151
Chapter 16	Collecting Specimens	153
Chapter 17	Measuring Vital Signs	156
Chapter 18	Special Procedures	158

PART 4   MEETING THE CLIENT'S SPECIAL NEEDS

Chapter 19	Caring for Older Adults	161
Chapter 20	Caring for Mothers, Infants, and Children	163
Chapter 21	Caring for Clients With Mental Illness	166
Chapter 22	Caring for Clients With Illnesses Requiring Home Care	168
Chapter 23	Caring for the Dying Client	171
Chapter 24	Emergencies	172

PART 5   PROFESSIONAL SKILLS

Chapter 25	Getting a Job and Keeping It	174

Skills Competency Checklists	177
Skills Competency Checklists Record	279

1

Part 1

Orientation to Home Care

Learning About Home Care

Matching

Directions: Match the terms listed in Column A with the correct definition in Column B.

COLUMN A

A. Ethnic
B. Client
C. Evaluation
D. Entry-level
E. Certification
F. Confidential
G. Role
H. Clinical experience

COLUMN B

1. _____ The usual function of a person
2. _____ The process of judging performance to determine progress in learning
3. _____ Beginning, just starting
4. _____ Practicing skills learned in the classroom in a client care setting under the supervision of the instructor or a home care nurse
5. _____ Person receiving care at home
6. _____ Recognition by a government or nongovernment agency that an individual has met certain requirements
7. _____ A group of people with the same origins or common traits
8. _____ Private information not to be discussed

Situations

Directions: Listed below are three situations about the home care training program. How would you respond? Discuss the answers in class.

SITUATION 1

Your friends are happy that you are starting a new career. They ask you to tell them all about your training program. In the space below, write what you would tell them about your home care training program.

RESPONSE:

Length of course _____

Clinical experience _____

Evaluations _____

SITUATION 2

Before you go to bed, you set out all the things you will need to take to class the next day. Your roommate wants to know why you are taking all these things (notebook, pen, pencils, and text-book) to class.

RESPONSE:

_____

_____

SITUATION 3

Your instructor uses some words that you do not understand. After class, your classmates complain that they don't know the meaning of those big words either.

RESPONSE:

_____

_____

Practicing to Take Tests

Directions: The following test questions give you a chance to sharpen your test-taking skills. Read each text item carefully, and then give the correct answer. Check your answer at the back of the book to see if your were right or wrong. Good luck.

EXAMPLES:
TRUE OR FALSE

Directions: In the space provided, mark the statement "T" for true or "F" for false. If false, change the statement to make it true.

1. _____ All home care aide training programs are the same number of hours in length.
2. _____ A person receiving home care is called a client.
3. _____ The PQRST method is a good way to study.
4. _____ The process of evaluating the home care aide's performance only occurs at the end of the program.
5. _____ The instructor is the only person who evaluates the student's ability to successfully work in the client's home.
6. _____ The ability of the home care aide to work cooperatively with classmates is an important part of being a successful student.

MULTIPLE CHOICE

Directions: Read carefully and select the best answer for each question. Circle the letter indicating the correct answer. There is only **one** correct answer for each question.

1. Clinical experience takes place:
   a. in the classroom.
   b. in the client's home.
   c. in your own home.
   d. wherever you are learning.

2. When reading the chapter in the textbook, a person should begin with:
   a. stories about clients.
   b. key terms.
   c. chapter objectives.
   d. study questions.

3. Written tests are an example of:
   a. classroom evaluation.
   b. clinical evaluation.
   c. your role.
   d. certification.

Real Life Situations

1. How many ethnic groups are represented in your class? Talk to two of your classmates who have a background different from you. Complete the following information:

	STUDENT #1	STUDENT #2
Country where they (or family) were born	_____	_____
Special foods they enjoy	_____	_____
Special events	_____	_____
Special customs	_____	_____
Languages they speak/understand	_____	_____

2. Plan a weekly schedule that shows the time you will spend studying or preparing assignments for class. Explain your plan to those you live with. Ask for their support.

2

The Home Care Industry

Matching

Directions: Match the terms listed in Column A with the correct definition in Column B.

Column A

A. Official agency
B. Medicaid
C. Chronic illness
D. Hospital discharge planner
E. Assess
F. Diagnostic related group (DRG)
G. Hospice
H. Reimbursement
I. Acute illness
J. Medicare
K. Standard
L. Policy, policies
M. Voluntary agency

Column B

1. _____ A listing of diagnoses used in establishing reimbursement by Medicare and Medicaid for hospitalization and medical care
2. _____ A federal program of hospitalization and health care insurance for persons over 65 and/or those with permanent disabilities
3. _____ A state and federal insurance program that pays for hospitalization and health care for low-income persons of all ages
4. _____ An illness with a rapid onset, severe symptoms, and of short length
5. _____ A disease showing little change, slow progress, and of long duration
6. _____ A program of care that assists the dying client to maintain a satisfactory lifestyle during the end stage of an illness
7. _____ A person who arranges for the care of a patient upon release from the hospital
8. _____ A gauge that is used as a basis for judgment
9. _____ To make payment for expense incurred
10. _____ To determine the client's needs for home care services
11. _____ A set of rules and regulations
12. _____ An agency sponsored by local or state government
13. _____ A nonprofit agency financed through tax-deductible contributions

Hidden Words—Qualities of a Home Care Aide

Directions: Find the hidden words listed below that describe the qualities of a home care aide. Hint: Words appear from top down or bottom up, across or backward, or crosswise. When you find the word, circle it and cross off the word in the list.

alert	courteous	patient
caring	dependable	pleasant
cheerful	enthusiastic	reliable
clean	honest	respectful
competent	kind	sincere
confident	neat	skillful
considerate	observant	willing
cooperative		

C	E	V	I	T	A	R	E	P	O	O	C	E	P
O	O	E	T	R	E	L	A	P	R	I	O	N	L
M	P	N	L	O	W	I	L	T	T	L	U	T	E
P	A	R	S	B	G	E	N	S	S	U	T	S	A
E	T	L	T	I	A	E	A	C	E	F	N	U	S
T	I	A	B	S	D	I	H	C	N	T	A	O	L
E	E	E	A	I	S	E	L	L	O	C	V	E	U
N	N	N	F	U	E	R	R	E	H	E	R	T	F
T	T	N	H	R	A	K	L	A	R	P	E	R	L
L	O	T	F	E	S	D	I	N	T	S	S	U	L
C	N	U	W	I	L	L	I	N	G	E	B	O	I
E	L	B	A	D	N	E	P	E	D	R	O	C	K
S	I	N	C	E	R	E	G	N	I	R	A	C	S

Word Completion

Directions: Name the team member who performs the following function:

FUNCTION	TEAM MEMBER
1. Teaches client helpful hints to improve swallowing	S _ _ _ _ _ T _ _ _ _ _ _ _ _
2. Coordinates activities of the team	C _ _ _ M _ _ _ _ _ _
3. Supervises the activities of the LPN/LVN and home care aide	R _ _ _ _ _ _ _ _ _ N _ _ _ _

   4. Gives spiritual guidance to the client   C _ _ _ _ _
   5. Instructs the client and family about preparing
      meals according to the diet ordered by the doctor   D _ _ _ _ _ _ _ _
   6. Checks breathing equipment being used by
      the client   R _ _ _ _ _ _ _ _ _ _ T _ _ _ _ _ _ _
   7. Arranges community services to be given   S _ _ _ _ _ W _ _ _ _ _
   8. Provides complex nursing care to clients with
      special needs   N _ _ _ _ S _ _ _ _ _ _ _ _
   9. Gives personal care to clients and performs light
      housekeeping duties   H _ _ _ C _ _ _ A _ _ _
  10. Assesses the client's ability to perform ADL   O _ _ _ _ _ _ _ _ _ _ T _ _ _ _ _ _ _
  11. Gives nursing care to clients whose conditions
      are stable   L _ _ _ _ _ _ _ P _ _ _ _ _ _ _ _ N _ _ _ _
  12. Teaches exercises to strengthen leg muscles   P _ _ _ _ _ _ _ T _ _ _ _ _ _ _ _

True or False

Directions: In the space proved, mark the statement "T" for true or "F" for false. If false, change the statement to make it true.

   1. _____ The needs of the client and family determine the kinds of members required on the home care team.
   2. _____ You develop an ear ache while you're at work. You may take your client's prescription drug provided you request permission.
   3. _____ The registered nurse is responsible for evaluating the client's progress of therapy given by the physical therapist.
   4. _____ After visitors arrive, sit down and talk with them.
   5. _____ It is the case manager's job to assess the kinds of services required for each client.
   6. _____ An example of client services provided by a community agency is home-delivered meals.
   7. _____ It isn't necessary to maintain healthy eating habits, provided you give good client care.
   8. _____ First impressions are usually lasting ones.
   9. _____ Your client's husband is drinking beer while he's eating lunch and offers you one, too. It's okay to have one beer, but not more.
  10. _____ The client's family asks you to work extra hours for which they will pay you. You agree, provided they do not notify the agency of this arrangement.

3

Developing Effective Communication Skills

True or False

Directions: In the space provided, mark the statement "T" for true or "F" for false. If false, change the statement to make it true.

1. _____ Hearing impaired persons will understand what you are saying if you exaggerate your words.
2. _____ It is helpful to keep a pad and pencil nearby so that your visually impaired client can communicate in writing, if necessary.
3. _____ Speak to the side where the client's hearing is better.
4. _____ Turn off the television and household appliances to reduce background noise before speaking to the hearing impaired client.
5. _____ Touching the visually impaired client's hand to get and keep attention is a good idea.
6. _____ Always stand to the side of visually impaired clients because their side vision is good.
7. _____ If possible, turn off exposed light bulbs and lower window shades to reduce glaring light when talking to your client who has poor vision.
8. _____ Speak in a loud tone of voice to make sure your blind client understands what you are saying.
9. _____ While your client, Mr. Jackson, is asking you a question, be sure to concentrate on how you will answer him.
10. _____ You know the answer to the question Maria Gonzales is asking, but you wait until she is finished talking before you respond.
11. _____ The client has the right to refuse treatment.
12. _____ The client has the right to refuse care given by an African American home care aide.
13. _____ Your client, who looks sad, is wearing heavy make-up that exaggerates her lips and eyebrows in an unbecoming way. You compliment her on how attractive she looks to make her feel better.

14. _____ The client has the right to know the plan of care, in advance.
15. _____ The home care aide has the right to be treated with respect and dignity by the client and family.

Situations

Directions: Listed below are three situations you may experience as a home care aide. How would you respond; what would you do? Discuss with your classmates.

SITUATION 1

You have been caring for your client, Sarah Walker, for several months. Her husband, Ben, has always been very friendly and compliments you on your appearance and quality of care each time you visit.

During your last visit, Ben asked you to go into the bedroom while Sarah was eating her breakfast in the kitchen. He said he wanted to talk about his wife's illness. He said, "I just want to talk to you alone. You are very special to me. I think you like me, too." Then, he reached for your hand.

RESPONSE:

_____

_____

_____

ACTION:

_____

_____

_____

SITUATION 2

This is the first day with your client, Joseph D'Orio, who is 87 years of age and very confused. He lives with his son, daughter-in-law, and two adult grandchildren.

While giving Mr. D'Orio a bath, you notice several bruises on his back and burn marks on his arms and legs. You ask Joseph about them, and he starts to cry. He says that his son doesn't love him anymore because he is such a burden.

RESPONSE:

_____

_____

_____

ACTION:

_____

_____

_____

SITUATION 3

You have been making daily visits to care for Amy Doyle, a disabled child who is 3 years of age. Each day for the last week, Amy's mother has been telling you how hard it is for her to pay for the rent, gas, electricity, and food.

Today, you arrive on the job and there is no heat or electricity in the apartment. Amy's mother asks you to call the gas company to have the services restored.

RESPONSE:

_____

_____

_____

ACTION:

_____

_____

_____

SITUATION 4

As you are putting on your coat to leave your client's apartment, her son, Harry, says "You have been very kind to my mother for these past six months and I really appreciate all that you have done for her. I just wanted you to have this—I know that it's not much, but we all can use some more cash during the holidays." Then he tries to put folded bills of money in your hand.

RESPONSE:

_____

_____

_____

ACTION:

_____

_____

_____

Matching

Directions: Match the terms in Column A with the correct definition in Column B

COLUMN A

A. Communication
B. Verbal communication
C. Nonverbal communication

D. Bias(es)

E. Prejudice
 F. Disability
G. Surrogate
H. Advance medical directive
 I. Grievance
 J. Confidentiality
K. Ethics

COLUMN B

1. _____ One who is appointed to act for another
2. _____ A wrong, considered as grounds for a formal complaint
3. _____ Sharing of thoughts, information, and opinions with others
4. _____ To like or dislike someone or something without a good reason
5. _____ Communication using the spoken or written word
6. _____ Code of behavior or conduct
7. _____ Physical, mental, or emotional condition that interferes with activities of daily living
8. _____ Something spoken or written in confidence, in secret
9. _____ Communication without the use of words
10. _____ Documents that indicate a client's wishes about health care
11. _____ Having or forming a preconceived judgment or opinion without fair reasons

Diagram

Directions: Label the diagram (Figure 3-1) using the terms listed below.

message
meaning
sender
receiver
feedback

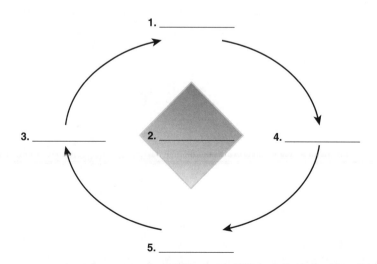

1. _____

3. _____   2. _____   4. _____

5. _____

Figure 3-1

Completion

Directions: Fill in the blanks after each question.

1. Effective communication begins with the basic principle _____

   _____

2. Five ways to improve listening skills are:

   a. _____

   b. _____

   c. _____

   d. _____

   e. _____

3. Two topics to avoid when communicating with your client are _____

   and _____.

4. Confidential information is shared with your supervisor when _____

   _____

5. To be a good listener, you must devote _____ to the
   speaker.

Understanding Your Client's Needs

Diagram

Directions: Label the pyramid (Figure 4-1) to show the basic human needs as described by Maslow. Use the words below and write in the appropriate space.

love
physical
self-actualization
security and safety
self-esteem

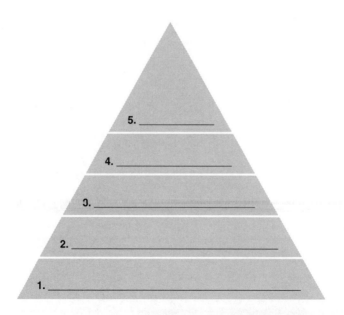

Figure 4-1

Completion

Directions: Complete the following statements.
1. Oxygen and food are examples of _____ need.
2. Preventing falls helps to meet a client's need for
_____
3. Feeling close to other persons helps to meet the need for
_____
4. Feeling good about oneself is meeting the need for
_____
5. By learning and creating, people meet their need for
_____

True or False

Directions: In the space provided, mark the statement "T" for true or "F" for false. If false, change the statement to make it true.
1. _____ We all belong to a nuclear family.
2. _____ Family means mother, father, and siblings.
3. _____ There is no typical family.
4. _____ Many families are mobile—moving from place to place.
5. _____ The most important structure in society is the family.
6. _____ Family members always work together to meet all of their own needs.
7. _____ The home care aide meets all the needs of the client and family.
8. _____ The needs of the client come first.
9. _____ Home care aides have no personal needs.
10. _____ When needs are unmet, physical and/or emotional problems can arise.

Growth and Development

Directions: List five principles of growth and development:
1. _____
2. _____
3. _____
4. _____
5. _____

Growth and Development Chart

Directions: Complete the chart below.

Development Stage	Age	Characteristics	Ways to Meet Client Needs
Infancy		1. Tremendous growth	1. Hold and cuddle
	to 1 year	2.	2.
		3.	3.
Toddler	1–3 years	1. Endless activity	1. Eliminate hazards
		2.	2.
		3.	3.
Preschool	____ years	1. Endless energy	1. Avoid use of "don't"
		2.	2.
		3.	3.
School age	6–12 years	1.	1.
		2.	2.
		3.	3.
Adolescent	____ years	1.	1.
		2.	2.
		3.	3.
Adulthood	18–65 years	1.	1.
		2.	2.
		3.	3.
Older adulthood	65–100+ years	1.	1.
		2.	2.
		3.	3.

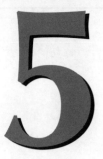

Understanding How the Body Works

Identification

Directions: In the space provided, identify the body system that contains the organ listed.

ORGAN   SYSTEM

1. pituitary gland   _____
2. liver   _____
3. prostate gland   _____
4. bronchioles   _____
5. diaphragm   _____
6. ribs   _____
7. arteries   _____
8. gallbladder   _____
9. capillaries   _____
10. ovaries   _____
11. urethra   _____
12. spinal cord   _____
13. larynx   _____
14. brain   _____

Fill in the Blanks

Directions: Beside the name of each body system, give its function.

BODY SYSTEM   FUNCTION

1. skeletal   _____
2. muscular   _____

   3. circulatory and lymphatic   _____
   4. integumentary   _____
   5. nervous   _____
   6. respiratory   _____
   7. endocrine   _____
   8. digestive   _____
   9. urinary   _____
  10. reproductive   _____

Matching

Directions: Match the definition in Column A with the correct term in Column B.

COLUMN A

A. Basic functioning unit of the body
B. Blood cells are produced here
C. The exchange of oxygen and carbon dioxide
   takes place here
D. Basic functioning unit of the kidney
E. Digestion of food is completed here
F. Stores urine
G. Secretions that enter the bloodstream from glands
H. Sends messages to other parts of the body
 I. The structure that sends food into the bloodstream
 J. Absorbs fluid back into the body

COLUMN B

 1. _____ villi
 2. _____ nephron
 3. _____ small intestine
 4. _____ nerves
 5. _____ hormones
 6. _____ large intestine
 7. _____ alveoli
 8. _____ long bones
 9. _____ bladder
10. _____ cell

Completion

Directions: Complete the following sentences by filling in the blanks.
   1. Tissues are made up of groups of _____.
   2. Another word for throat is _____.
   3. Arteries carry blood _____ the heart.
   4. _____ connect arteries to veins.
   5. A heart beat has two parts: _____ and _____.
   6. A body system is made up of many _____.
   7. Another word for windpipe is _____.
   8. The lid that prevents food from entering the respiratory system is the _____.
   9. The long, strong muscles are in the _____.
  10. The urethra has two functions in the man because it carries _____
      and _____.

Diagram

Directions: Fill in the blanks beside each figure (Figures 5-1 to 5-3).

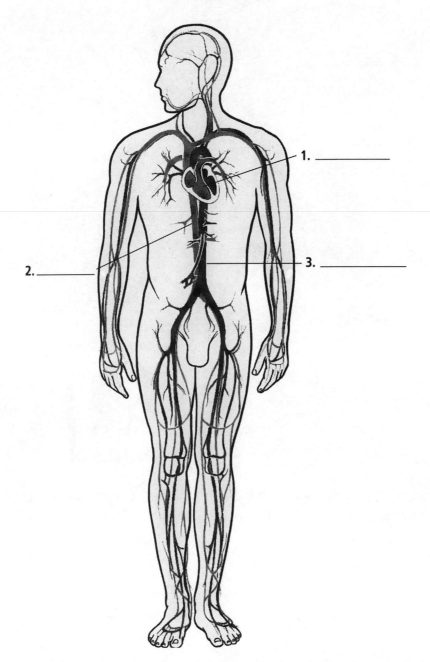

1. _____

2. _____

3. _____

Figure 5-1 *(From Thibodeau GA, Patton KT:* Anatomy and Physiology, *ed 4, St. Louis, 1999, Mosby.)*

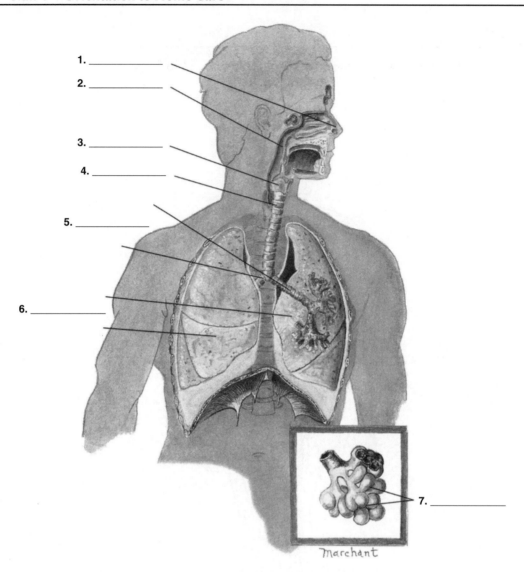

1. _____

2. _____

3. _____

4. _____

5. _____

6. _____

7. _____

Figure 5-2 *(From Sorrentino SA, Gorek B:* Mosby's Textbook for Long-Term Care Assistants, *ed 3, St. Louis, 1999, Mosby.)*

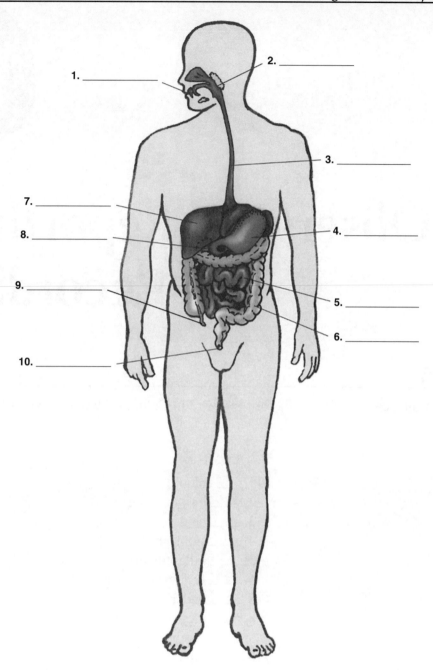

Figure 5-3 *(From Thibodeau GA, Patton KT:* Anatomy and Physiology, *ed 4, St. Louis, 1999, Mosby.)*

6

Observing, Reporting, and Recording

Matching

Directions: Match each prefix, suffix, or root word in Column A with the correct definition in Column B.

COLUMN A

A. -itis
B. gastro-
C. arthro-
D. -uria
E. -ostomy
F. cerebro-
G. hyper-
H. post-
I. -ectomy
J. hemo-
K. hypo-
L. -algia

COLUMN B

1. _____ blood
2. _____ new opening
3. _____ pain
4. _____ stomach
5. _____ inflammation
6. _____ surgical removal
7. _____ under
8. _____ urine or urination
9. _____ cerebrum
10. _____ joint
11. _____ above
12. _____ after

Reporting and Recording

Directions: Beside each observation, indicate the action you would take in reporting and recording the information.

1. Bruise on client's arm   _____
2. Client complains of sudden pain in chest   _____
3. Foul odor in refrigerator   _____
4. Severe difficulty in breathing   _____

5. Sudden vomiting and diarrhea _____
6. Toilet overflowed—client lives alone; has no immediate family nearby _____
7. Client refused lunch and drank one cup of tea _____
8. Client cried for half hour after brother's visit _____
9. Client's daughter slapped her twice in the face during 15-minute visit _____
10. Client had been irritable but now is pleasant and talkative _____

True or False

Directions: In the space provided, mark the statement "T" for true or "F" for false. If false, change the statement to make it true.

1. ____ Client care records are permanent, written, legal documents.
2. ____ The care record can be shared with family members.
3. ____ The entire care record is kept in the client's home.
4. ____ Home care aides usually chart on a check list.
5. ____ Client care records may be used as evidence in court cases.
6. ____ Always use a pen when writing on a client record.
7. ____ Change the care plan if you believe that it is necessary.
8. ____ Vital signs are temperature, pulse, respirations, and blood pressure.
9. ____ The agency should be notified whenever you observe changes in the client's physical condition or mental condition.
10. ____ Don't call your supervisor too much; you shouldn't be a pest.

Abbreviations

Directions: Give the meanings for the following abbreviations:

1. abd _____
2. ADL _____
3. BP _____
4. Ca _____
5. meds _____
6. O_2 _____
7. OOB _____
8. ROM _____
9. Tbsp _____
10. TPR _____
11. $\bar{c}$ _____
12. ml _____
13. $\bar{s}$ _____
14. tsp _____

Recording

Directions: Complete the client care record (Figure 6-1, "Change in Condition" section on p. 25) for the following:

Ten minutes after you arrive at your client's home (9:10 A.M.), she vomits her breakfast. She complains of feeling dizzy; her skin is bluish, and her breathing is noisy. You call 9-1-1, your supervisor, and your client's sister who is upstairs. Your client is taken to the medical center by the ambulance at 9:45 A.M. Her sister goes with her. Your supervisor comes to the home.

Checklist

Directions: Complete a client care record (Figure 6-1) for the following:

OOB to chair
assist with shower and dressing
change and make bed

wash, dry, and fold personal laundry/linens
clean client bathroom
weigh daily before shower

Situation

Directions: Complete answers to the following situation:

Your client, Mr. Leo, tells you that he has "indigestion." He says, "It must be from the fried eggs and sausage I had for breakfast." He asks you to get his "indigestion medicine."

List three actions you should take:

1. _____
2. _____
3. _____

Incident Report

Directions: Complete an incident report (Figure 6-2 on p. 26) for the following situation:

When you step onto the porch at your client's home, your left foot goes through a weak board. You fall, scrape your left leg, and hurt your left ankle, which becomes swollen and painful. You limp into the client's home and call your supervisor. He comes over to assess your injury, takes you to the emergency room for treatment, and completes an incident report.

WEEKLY CLIENT CARE RECORD

Client _____ Employee _____

Address _____ Title _____

City _____ State ____ Zip _____ Soc. Sec. No. _____

Phone (day) _____ (eve.) _____ Week Ending _____ / _____ / _____

Fill in the date for each day.

Write your initials in the box which corresponds to each task performed.

	DATE							
DAY		Mon.	Tue.	Wed.	Th.	Fri.	Sat.	Sun.
TIME ARRIVED								

PERSONAL CARE:

Bath ❑ Bed ❑ Chair ❑ Shower ❑ Tub								
Perineal Care								
Hair ❑ Groom ❑ Shampoo								
Mouthcare ❑ Denture Care								
Shave								
Nail Care ❑ Clean ❑ File								
Foot Care								
Special Skin Care								
Dressing ❑ Assist ❑ Complete								
Toileting ❑ Bed Pan ❑ Commode ❑ BRP								
Other instructions: _____								

CLIENT ACTIVITIES:

Transfer Activity Instructions: _____

Assist with walking ❑ Cane ❑ Walker ❑ Crutches								
Assist with exercises ❑ ROM ❑ Other (specify)								
Wheelchair activities								
Other instructions: _____								

Figure 6-1

(continued)	Mon.	Tue.	Wed.	Th.	Fri.	Sat.	Sun.
OTHER FUNCTIONS:							
Temp. ❑ Oral ❑ Rectal ❑ Underarm ❑ Ear							
Pulse							
Respirations							
Blood Pressure							
Weigh Client							
Record Intake/Output (use special form)							
OTHER FUNCTIONS:							
Prepare and serve meal/snack							
Special diet (Specify)							
Assist with feeding							
Medications reminder							
Stoma care							
Incontinent care							
Record bowel movements							
Change in condition (use special form section)							
Other instructions:							
HOUSEHOLD SERVICES:							
Change/make client's bed							
Clean client's room							
Clean bathroom							
Clean kitchen; wash dishes							
Vacuum, sweep, dust							
Client laundry							
Marketing							
Errands (specify) _____							
Other instructions: _____							
DEPARTURE TIME							
TOTAL HOURS							

I certify that the hours shown represent my true total hours worked.

Signature _____ Title _____ Date _____

Return form to Home Care Agency weekly.
Notify Home Care Agency if your client's condition has changed since your last visit.

Figure 6-1 (*Continued*)

WEEKLY CLIENT CARE RECORD—CHANGE IN CONDITION

Date	Time	Observation	Action Taken

Signed:
_____

Figure 6-1 (*Continued*)

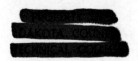

ABC Home Care Agency
INCIDENT REPORT

PERSON INVOLVED	(Last name)	(First name)	(Middle initial)						
Address				Adult ☐	Child ☐	Male ☐	Female ☐	Age ___	

Date of incident/accident	Time of incident/accident	A.M. ☐ P.M. ☐	Exact location of incident/accident
			Bedroom ☐ Hallway ☐ Bathroom ☐ Other ☐ Specify ___

CLIENT ☐ List diagnosis if contributed to incident/accident:

Client's condition before incident/accident
Normal ☐   Confused ☐   Disoriented ☐   Sedated ☐ (Drug___ Dose___ Time___)   Other ☐ Specify ___

Were bed rails ordered? Yes ☐ No ☐
Were bed rails present? Yes ☐ No ☐
If Yes, Up ☐ Down ☐
Was height of bed adjustable? Yes ☐ No ☐
If Yes, Up ☐ Down ☐

EMPLOYEE ☐   Name ___   Job title ___   Length of time in this position ___

VISITOR ☐
OTHER ☐
Home address ___   Home phone ___
Occupation ___   Reason for presence ___

Equipment involved ☐
Property involved ☐   Describe ___
Was person authorized to be at location of incident/accident? Yes ☐ No ☐

Describe exactly what happened; why it happened; what the causes were. If injury, state part of body injured. If property ot equipment damaged, describe damage.

Indicate on diagram location of injury:

Temp. ___   Pulse. ___   Resp. ___
B.P. ___

TYPE OF INJURY
1. Laceration ☐
2. Hematoma ☐
3. Abrasion ☐
4. Burn ☐
5. Swelling ☐
6. None apparent ☐
7. Other (specify below) ☐

LEVEL OF CONSCIOUSNESS

Name of supervisor notified	Time of notification ___ A.M./P.M.	Time of responded ___ A.M./P.M.
Name and relationship of family member notified	Time of notification ___ A.M./P.M.	Time of responded ___ A.M./P.M.

Was person involved seen by a physician? Yes ☐ No ☐ If Yes, physician's name | Where | Date | Time A.M.☐ P.M.☐
Was first aid administered? Yes ☐ No ☐ If Yes, type of provided by whom | Where | Date | Time A.M.☐ P.M.☐
Was person involved taken to a hospital? Yes ☐ No ☐ If Yes, hospital name | By whom | Date | Time A.M.☐ P.M.☐

Name, title (if applicable), address & phone no. of witness(es) | Additional comments and/or steps taken to prevent recurrence:

SIGNATURE/TITLE/DATE | **SIGNATURE/TITLE/DATE**
Person preparing report | Case Manager
Supervisor | Administrator

INCIDENT REPORT

Figure 6-2 *(Modified from Briggs Corporation, Des Moines, Iowa.)*

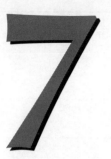

Working With the Ill and Disabled

Client Reactions

Directions: Read the following client situations. In the space provided, identify the client's reaction and explain what you would do.

1. Hector, who is able to feed himself, has finished half of his meal. You observe that he has had difficulty today controlling his fork. Therefore you suggest that he use a spoon to finish eating his food. Suddenly, Hector takes the fork and throws it across the room.

   A. Hector is showing:

   _____

   B. What would you do?

   _____
   _____
   _____
   _____

2. You enter Rita's bedroom to begin preparing for her bed bath. She does not respond to your greeting and turns her back toward you as you speak to her.

   A. Rita's reaction is called:

   _____

   B. What would you do?

   _____
   _____
   _____
   _____

3. Maria has weak leg muscles, and the physical therapist has instructed her to perform exercises each day. When you ask her to show you how she exercises, she says, "I really don't think

I can do them. What will happen if I fall? I'm so weak." Then she wrings her hands and shakes her head "No."

A. Maria's response shows:

_____

B. What would you do?

_____

_____

4. Sam is being cared for by his wife who says she does "everything" for him. Your supervisor has given you instructions to encourage Sam to perform activities of daily living (ADL). When you give him the washcloth to clean his face, he says, "You wash me. My wife always does it for me."

A. Sam is demonstrating:

_____

B. What would you do?

_____

_____

5. Robert has diabetes and is on a severely restricted diet of sugars. You prepare his lunch according to the food requirements ordered by the doctor. He says the food you prepare is Okay but he "likes lots of sweets." His daughter tells you that he hides candy in his bedroom and eats it when he's watching television at night. His response to why he eats all that candy is, "It won't hurt me. I know the doctor made a mistake—I'm not a diabetic."

A. Robert's response shows:

_____

B. What would you do?

_____

_____

Family Situations

Directions: Read the following family situations. In the space provided, answer the question given for each situation.

1. Mrs. Tucker tells you that she feels like everything she does for her husband is "all wrong." He is nasty, complains, and wants things right away. Mr. Tucker has been ill for the past 5 years and is becoming increasingly unable to perform ADL. His wife says, "I am so tired, so hurt, and so disgusted! I just don't know what to do. I could sit here and cry all day." As the home care aide, what could you do to help the Tucker family?

_____

_____

2. Ann Marie Burroughs is a high school student aged 17 years who was diagnosed with cancer of the bone. Her leg was amputated above the knee. After the surgery, she is at home waiting for her artificial limb to be delivered and fitted. Meanwhile, she is crutch-walking using the

remaining limb. You are helping with her personal care at home—bathing, grooming, and other ADL. Ann Marie spends most of her day crying. She will not see any of her friends, does not answer the telephone, and refuses to work with the home teacher. Ann Marie says her life is over, she might as well be dead, and she is never going back to school or out of the house again. Her mother is very concerned and asks you what can be done to help.

_____

_____

_____

3. Jose Santiago, aged 36 years, has to care for both of his parents, aged 72 years. His father has had a stroke, is paralyzed on one side of the body, and is unable to care for himself. Mrs. Santiago fell and fractured her hip. She uses a walker and needs assistance with personal care and grooming. Jose is doing all of the housekeeping, shopping, and cooking. He says that he has no income during this period and that things are really getting tough. His parents' Social Security checks don't seem to go far enough, and the rent, utility bills, car payment, and auto insurance are all due. Jose tells you that he is very anxious because he needs to work, yet his parents need his help and care, too. What would you do to help the Santiago family?

_____

_____

_____

_____

Crossword Puzzle

Directions: Complete the crossword puzzle by identifying important terms found in Chapter 7.

Crossword Puzzle

ACROSS

1. Avoids contact with others
4. Feeling of intense sadness
6. Duties and responsibilities assumed by a person
7. A refusal to admit the truth
8. Loss of ability to perform function(s)
10. State of relying too much on others

DOWN

2. Feeling very mad
3. A state of physical, mental, and social well-being
5. Absence of health
9. State of intense worry and/or fear

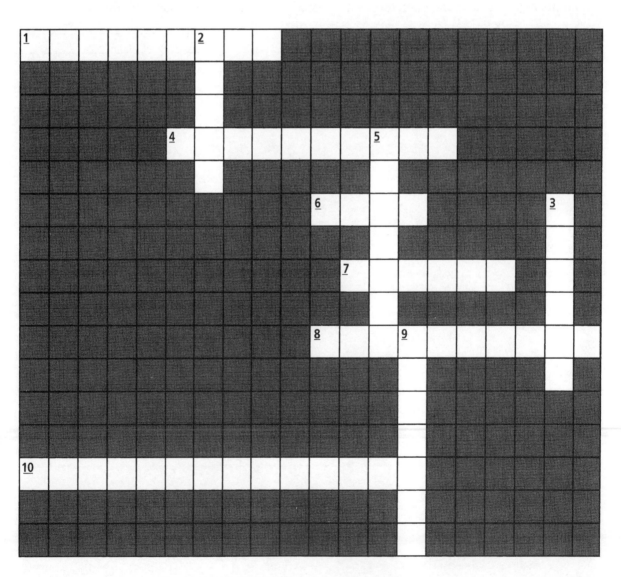

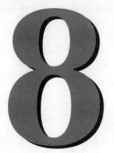

Part 2

Managing the Home Environment

Maintaining a Safe Environment

Home Hazards

Directions: In the picture below (Figure 8-1) there are more than 10 safety hazards. In the space provided, list 10 hazards and a safety measure to correct each.

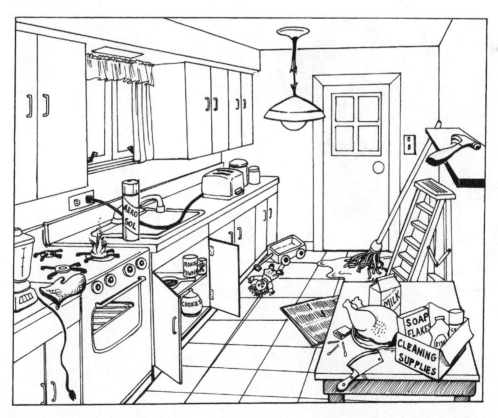

Figure 8-1

31

HAZARDS

1. _____
2. _____
3. _____
4. _____
5. _____
6. _____
7. _____
8. _____
9. _____
10. _____

SAFETY MEASURE

1. _____
2. _____
3. _____
4. _____
5. _____
6. _____
7. _____
8. _____
9. _____
10. _____

Diagram

Directions: Label the diagram below (Figure 8-2) to show the three ingredients that combine to start a fire. Give two examples of each.

1. _____

3. _____   2. _____

1. _____
   _____
2. _____
   _____
3. _____
   _____

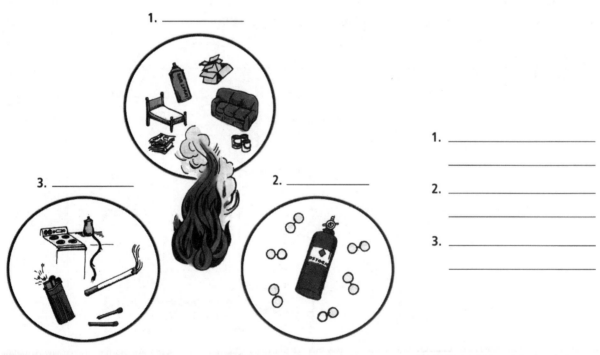

Figure 8-2

Matching

Directions: Match each item in Column A with one of the ingredients to start a fire from Column B.

COLUMN A		COLUMN B
1. Cigarettes	_____	A. Fuel
2. Pilot light	_____	B. Oxygen
3. Clothing	_____	C. Heat source
4. Air	_____	
5. Cigarette lighter	_____	
6. Medical oxygen	_____	
7. Elevator shaft	_____	
8. Pot holders	_____	
9. Open doors leading to fire exits	_____	
10. Frayed electrical cord	_____	
11. Oily rags	_____	
12. Stacks of old newspapers	_____	

Situations

Directions: Read each situation. Answer the questions in the space provided.

1. Willie Mae Jones takes the bus to get to and from her client's eighth floor apartment in the city. The bus stop is two blocks from her home. She then walks three more blocks to reach her client's apartment house. This area has many small stores that are open for business during the day but are closed when she gets the 6 P.M. bus to go home.

   A. List three personal safety rules Willie Mae should use when walking to/from the bus stop and waiting for the bus.
      1. _____
      2. _____
      3. _____

   B. List three safety rules when riding the bus.
      1. _____
      2. _____
      3. _____

   C. List three safety precautions she needs to take before reaching the door to her client's apartment or her own home.
      1. _____
      2. _____
      3. _____

2. Ethel's client lives on a farm. She uses her own car to travel 20 miles from her home to the farm house. There are no gas stations on this route, one roadside restaurant, and only two houses, located $1/2$ mile back from the road. Ethel is concerned about her safety while traveling this rural road, especially after dark. In the space below give eight safety rules you would encourage Ethel to use while traveling to and from her client's home.

1. _____
2. _____
3. _____
4. _____
5. _____
6. _____
7. _____
8. _____

3. You have been asked to gather ideas for a disaster supply kit. Of the items listed below, select those you would use in preparing the kit by placing a "Yes" or "No" in the space provided.

_____ Blanket
_____ Eating utensils
_____ Pots and pans
_____ Money, including coins
_____ First aid kit
_____ Extra car keys
_____ Flashlight, including batteries
_____ Important papers (e.g., insurance policies, wills)
_____ Essential medications in childproof containers
_____ Sweater
_____ Canned food and can opener
_____ Bottle of liquor
_____ Bottle of water
_____ Shampoo
_____ Hairspray

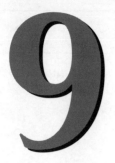

Maintaining a Healthy Environment

Household Tasks Schedule

Directions: In the space next to each household task, write whether it should be performed weekly or daily.

Making client's bed   _____
Cleaning refrigerator   _____
Cleaning commode   _____
Changing bed linens   _____
Removing trash   _____
Laundering bed linens   _____
Picking up clutter   _____
Washing dishes   _____
Dusting living room   _____
Cleaning toilet and bathroom sink   _____
Sweeping kitchen floor   _____
Cleaning kitchen counters   _____

Cleaning and Storing Supplies

Directions: Describe the care of the following items after each use.

Dust cloths   _____
Broom   _____
Sponges   _____
Bucket   _____
Toilet brush   _____
Rubber utility gloves _____

Sorting Laundry

Directions: The items of clothing listed in the left column below need to be sorted into washer loads. For each item, select the correct type of load needed.

_____	1. Dirty work clothes	A. Sturdy white
_____	2. White cotton athletic socks	B. Dark
_____	3. Blue toilet lid cover	C. Colorfast
_____	4. Cotton print sheets	D. Heavily soiled
_____	5. Nylon underwear	E. Delicate
_____	6. White cotton sheets	
_____	7. Blue jeans	
_____	8. Light purple towels	
_____	9. Dark brown cotton tee shirt	
_____	10. Yellow jogging top and pants	
_____	11. Diapers	
_____	12. Pink embroidered sweater	

True or False

Directions: In the space provided, mark the statement "T" for true or "F" for false. If false, change the statement to make it true.

1. _____ Sick people are not able to care for their own homes.
2. _____ The client's physical needs come before housekeeping duties.
3. _____ Always work from the cleanest to the dirtiest area.
4. _____ Use a bag or basket to collect clutter.
5. _____ Use a sharp knife to remove frost from the refrigerator freezer.
6. _____ Wash wooden bowls in the automatic dishwasher.
7. _____ Use baking soda solution to clean the refrigerator.
8. _____ When treating linens stained with body fluids, wear gloves.
9. _____ Never mix chlorine bleach with ammonia.
10. _____ Do not make comments about your client's poor housekeeping.
11. _____ Wear protective gloves when using household cleaning solutions.
12. _____ Read the care label before washing clothes.

10

Meeting the Client's Nutritional Needs

Fill in the Blank

Directions: Fill in the missing words on the blank lines for each statement.

1. Food energy is measured by means of a unit called a _____.
2. Carbohydrates are composed of the chemicals _____, _____, and _____.
3. Sugars and starches are examples of _____.
4. Amino acids are components of _____.
5. Vitamins A, D, E, and K are _____ vitamins.
6. A tool to use in menu planning is the _____.
7. Adults should eat _____ servings of food from the bread, cereal, rice, and pasta group.
8. Too much saturated fat may raise the level of _____ in the blood.
9. Roughage is another word for _____.
10. The term used to describe poor appetite is _____.
11. When assisting a blind client to eat, the plate is described as a _____.
12. Foods high in salt are eliminated on the _____ restricted diet.
13. Spicy, highly seasoned, and fried foods are omitted in the _____ diet.
14. The human body is _____ percent fluid.
15. The daily need for water (fluids) is at least _____.
16. Lack of fluid in the body can cause _____.
17. Three factors to consider in menu planning are _____, _____, and _____.
18. Butter, cream, and ice cream would be omitted on a _____ diet.
19. Proper storage is essential to preserve the _____ and _____ of foods.
20. Calcium and phosphorus are examples of _____ found in food and needed by the human body.

Crossword Puzzle

Directions: Complete the crossword puzzle by identifying important terms found in Chapter 10.

ACROSS

1. Microorganisms that cause disease
3. High grade, superior
4. Having excessive water loss from body tissues
6. Nourishment

DOWN

2. A disorder of nutrition
5. A lack of one or more nutrients from diet
7. A method of pricing food

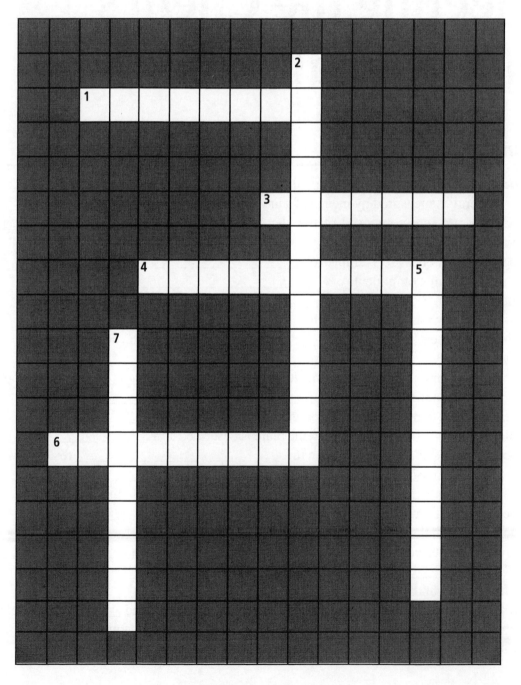

Food Guide Pyramid

Directions: Complete the pyramid (Figure 10-1) by filling in the food groups and the recommended servings for each.

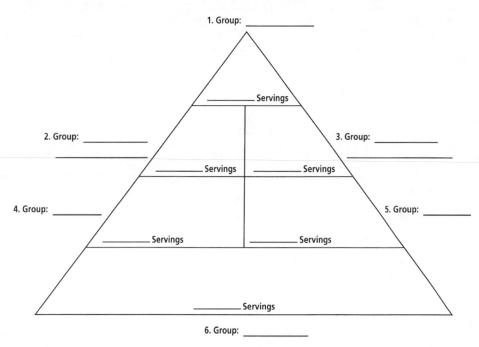

1. Group: _____

_____ Servings

2. Group: _____
_____

3. Group: _____
_____

_____ Servings   _____ Servings

4. Group: _____

5. Group: _____

_____ Servings   _____ Servings

_____ Servings

6. Group: _____

Figure 10-1

Matching

Directions: Match the eating problems listed in Column A with ways to prepare clients' meals listed in Column B. There may be more than one correct match.

COLUMN A

A. Low energy levels
B. Difficulty chewing
C. Difficulty swallowing
D. Poor appetite

COLUMN B

1. _____ Avoid serving crackers
2. _____ Prepare attractive, colorful meals
3. _____ Use drinking straws
4. _____ Avoid celery stalks and raw carrots
5. _____ Serve thick, soft foods
6. _____ Cut food into small pieces
7. _____ Use thickeners in fluids
8. _____ Use lightweight cups, glassware
9. _____ Serve fluids about 1 hour before meals
10. _____ Cut meat, butter bread
11. _____ Prepare small meals and snacks
12. _____ Add gelatin to cold liquids
13. _____ Allow plenty of time to eat

Therapeutic Diets

Directions: Change the regular diet menu in Column A to meet the requirements for the diets listed above Columns B, C, and D (Figure 10-2).

A	B	C	D
REGULAR	HIGH FIBER	LOW SODIUM	LOW FAT/ CHOLESTEROL
Canned or Homemade Soup			
Ham Sandwich on Bread			
Mayonnaise			
Lettuce and Tomato			
Whole Milk			
Cookies			

Figure 10-2

Situations

Directions: Listed below are three situations you may experience as a home care aide. In the space provided, give the information requested.
1. Your client has prepared the following shopping list. To use it, indicate, beside each item, what additional information you will need.
   Milk _____
   Bread _____
   Orange juice _____
   Eggs _____
   Chopped beef _____
   Carrots _____
   Bananas _____
   Broccoli _____
   Toilet paper _____
   Ice cream _____
2. When you return from purchasing the items listed above, they must be stored properly. Where will you store them to preserve quality and/or maintain freshness?
   Milk _____
   Bread _____
   Orange juice _____

Eggs   _____

Chopped beef   _____

Carrots   _____

Bananas   _____

Broccoli   _____

Toilet paper   _____

Ice cream   _____

3. Your client, Mrs. Smith, tells you that she wants to go to the new food warehouse to see whether the prices are cheaper than the supermarket. She tells you to put her wheelchair in the back of your car and drive her there. What is your response? What would you do?

Response: _____

Action: _____

Part 3
Home Care Procedures

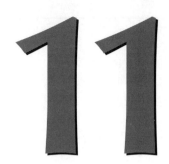

Preventing Infection/ Medical Asepsis

Matching

Directions: Match the terms in Column A with the correct definition in Column B.

COLUMN A

A. Standard (universal) precautions
B. Pathogenic
C. Disinfection
D. Host
E. Carrier
F. Sterile
G. Personal protective equipment
H. Exposure incident
I. Bloodborne pathogen
J. Medical asepsis
K. Infection
L. Nonpathogenic

COLUMN B

1. _____ Free from all living organisms
2. _____ Specialized clothing or equipment worn by an employee for protection against a biohazard
3. _____ Process that destroys pathogenic organisms
4. _____ Occurs when harmful organisms enter the body and grow, causing illness or disease
5. _____ Rules to follow to prevent bloodborne disease
6. _____ A person or animal in which microorganisms live
7. _____ Pathogenic microorganisms that are present in human blood and can cause disease in humans
8. _____ Usually not capable of causing or producing a disease
9. _____ Capable of causing a disease
10. _____ Situation when client's blood may enter the health care worker's body
11. _____ A person or animal that spreads disease to others but does not become ill
12. _____ Use of techniques and practices to prevent the spread of pathogenic organisms

True or False

Directions: In the space provided, mark the statement "T" for true or "F" for false. If false, change the statement to make it true.

1. _____ Always wear gloves when cleaning up blood spills.
2. _____ Standard (universal) precautions should be taken only if your client has Acquired Immunodeficiency Syndrome (AIDS).
3. _____ When in doubt about disinfecting items in the home, ask the client.
4. _____ Wash your hands after removing gloves.
5. _____ Microorganisms are found only in the human body.
6. _____ The person's skin acts as a natural defense against infection.
7. _____ OSHA regulations concerning bloodborne pathogens must be followed by doctors and nurses only.
8. _____ When masks or gowns become wet, they are no longer effective barriers to pathogens.
9. _____ Three signs of infection are pain, swelling, and redness of the area.
10. _____ Remove rings before applying gloves.

Completion

Directions: Fill in the missing words on the blank line(s) for each statement.

1. To grow and multiply, all microorganisms need_____, _____, and _____; or _____, _____, and _____.
2. Boil items for _____ minutes to destroy pathogenic organisms.
3. When preparing vinegar solution, use _____ part vinegar to _____ parts water.
4. Disinfection using the oven requires that items be baked for _____ at a temperature of _____ °F (_____ °C).
5. When preparing bleach solution, use _____ part bleach to _____ parts water.
6. Bleach solution must be put in a plastic container. The label must contain this information: _____, _____, and _____.
7. Handwashing is required _____ giving client care and _____ giving client care.
8. The most common household disinfecting solution is _____ or _____ and _____ _____.
9. Microorganisms can be transmitted by means of _____, _____, _____, _____ or _____ human contact, _____, _____.
10. Factors that help to increase the risk for infectious diseases include:
    a. _____
    b. _____
    c. _____
    d. _____
    e. _____

Situations

Directions: In the space provided, answer the questions for each situation.

1. As you remove the linens from your client's bed, you are stuck by an uncapped needle on an insulin syringe that has been accidentally left in the bed. What would you do?

_____
_____
_____

2. Mr. Werts is coughing up sputum and spitting it into an old coffee can. He wants you to empty the can into the toilet and return it to him. What would you do?

_____
_____
_____
_____

3. Mrs. Hunt uses two disposable insulin syringes a day. She also uses four lancets (short pointed blades) to collect blood to test her sugar level. How would Mrs. Hunt safely discard these "sharps"?

_____
_____
_____
_____

4. Your client has had an "accident" in bed. The client, his clothing, and the linens are soiled with urine and feces. Describe:
Protective equipment you would use:

_____
_____
_____
_____

How you would transport soiled clothing and linen to the laundry area in the basement of the home:

_____
_____
_____

How you would pretreat and launder soiled linens:

_____
_____
_____
_____
_____

Cycle of Infection

Directions: Label the six parts of the cycle of infection in the drawing below (Figure 11-1).

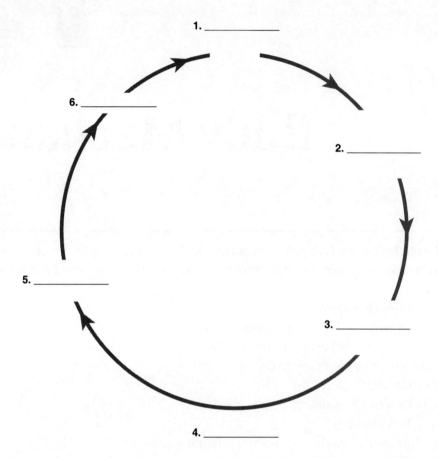

Figure 11-1

12

Body Mechanics

Procedures

Directions: Listed below are five procedures (including six major steps for each) used to assist clients to move in and out of bed. For each procedure, review the steps listed and number them in the correct order.

1. Applying a transfer (gait) belt
   _____ Apply belt over clothing and around waist.
   _____ Place belt buckles off center in front or back.
   _____ Explain what you are going to do.
   _____ Wash your hands.
   _____ Assist client to sit on side of bed.
   _____ Tighten belt until it is snug.

2. Transferring from bed to chair/wheelchair—standing transfer
   _____ Lock brakes and place footrests out of the way.
   _____ Wash your hands.
   _____ Assist client to sit at side of bed.
   _____ Have client reach back and grasp the farthest armrest of the wheelchair with one hand, then the nearest armrest.
   _____ Place wheelchair parallel to bed on client's strong side.
   _____ Place your arms under client's arms and around client's back, locking fingers together.

3. Assisting client to sit on side of bed
   _____ Provide privacy.
   _____ Assist client to put on robe and footwear.
   _____ Lock wheels on bed or push bed against wall if there are no brakes.
   _____ Place client in Fowler's position.
   _____ On count of "3", shift your weight to back leg and slowly swing client's legs over edge of bed while pulling shoulders to sitting position.
   _____ Explain what you are going to do.

4. Raising client's head and shoulders
   ____ Explain what you are going to do.
   ____ Slip your farthest arm under client's neck and shoulders.
   ____ Rock client to a semisitting position.
   ____ Wash your hands.
   ____ Lower head of bed and remove pillows.
   ____ Lock arms with client on side nearest you.
5. Moving client to side of bed
   ____ Explain what you are going to do.
   ____ Place arms underneath client.
   ____ Move client in three segments from center of bed to the edge.
   ____ Stand with feet apart.
   ____ Shift weight from front leg to back leg when moving client.
   ____ Wash your hands.

Identify the Incorrect Posture

Directions: What is wrong with the following pictures (Figures 12-1, 12-2, and 12-3)? In the space provided, explain how you would correct the picture.

1. (Figure 12-1) _____
   _____
   _____
   _____
   _____
   _____

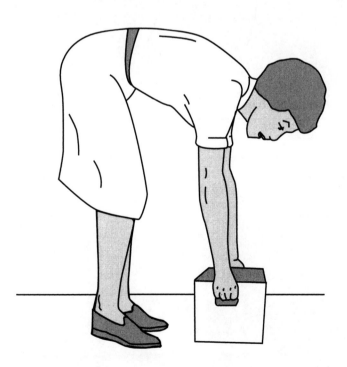

Figure 12-1

2. (Figure 12-2) _____
_____
_____
_____
_____
_____

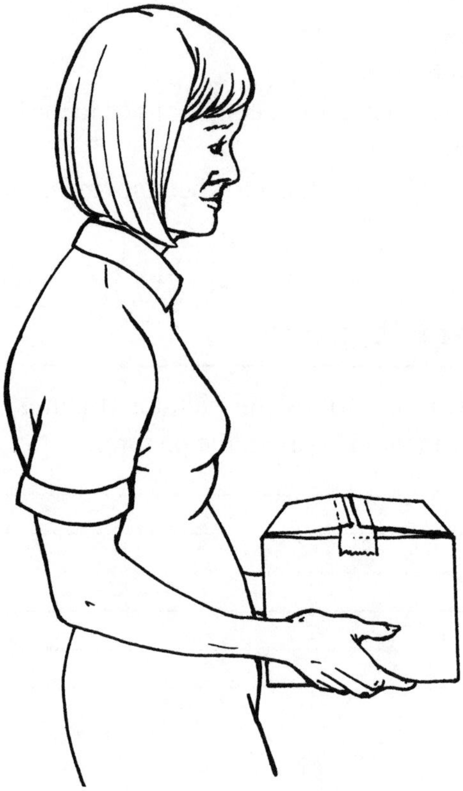

Figure 12-2

3. (Figure 12-3) _____
_____
_____
_____
_____
_____

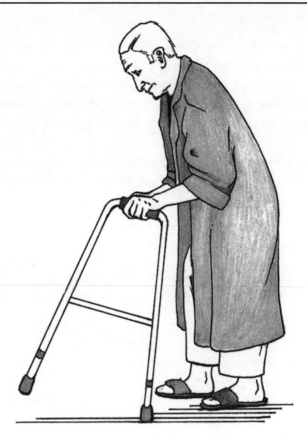

Figure 12-3

Matching

Directions: Match the terms listed in Column A with the correct definition in Column B.

COLUMN A

A. Body mechanics
B. Shearing
C. Contractures
D. Bed cradle
E. Ambulate
F. Pressure ulcer
G. Fatigue
H. Pneumonia
I. Walker
J. Immobility

COLUMN B

1. ＿＿ to walk
2. ＿＿ example of assistive device
3. ＿＿ device to keep weight of upper bedding off client's feet and legs
4. ＿＿ loss of ability to move
5. ＿＿ pressure against surface of skin and skin layers as client is being moved
6. ＿＿ proper use of muscles to move and lift objects
7. ＿＿ inflammation of the lung
8. ＿＿ muscles shorten and joints become permanently immovable
9. ＿＿ loss of strength and endurance
10. ＿＿ sore on the skin caused by prolonged pressure on the part (bed sore)

Situations

Directions: Read the following situations and answer the questions for each.

1. This is your first visit to Mr. Rand, a man aged 65 years who is recovering from surgery to repair a fractured hip. The physical therapist has been instructing him on exercises to strengthen the leg and arm muscles. His girlfriend usually helps him to get out of bed to practice his exercises. During your visit, you explain how he can help you as you assist him to get out of bed. He responds, "Oh, no, that's not how my girlfriend does it." The girlfriend then tells you how she helps him, which is not correct and is unsafe for both Mr. Rand and his girlfriend. What would you do?

   _____

   _____

   _____

2. As your client walks from her living room to the kitchen, she complains of dizziness and begins to fall. You ease her to the floor. She complains of feeling faint and weak. What would your next action be?

   _____

   _____

   _____

   _____

Identify the Position

Directions: Write the name of the position next to each figure (Figures 12-4 through 12-8).

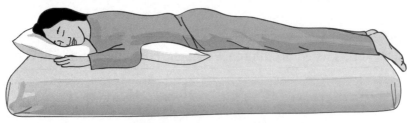

Figure 12-4

1. _____

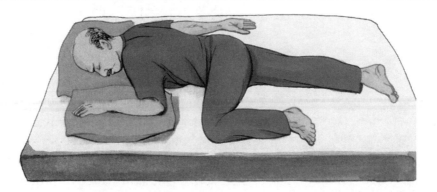

Figure 12-5

2. _____

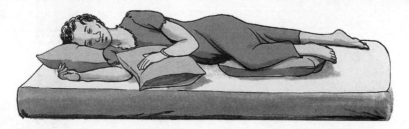

Figure 12-6

3. _____

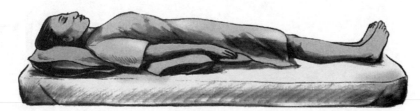

Figure 12-7

4. _____

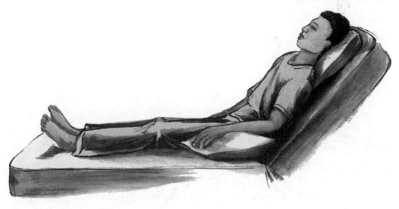

Figure 12-8

5. _____

Safety Factors

Directions: List 10 safety factors to consider when positioning, moving, and/or lifting clients.

1. _____
2. _____
3. _____
4. _____
5. _____
6. _____
7. _____
8. _____
9. _____
10. _____

13

Bedmaking

Diagram

Directions: In the space provided, identify the linens used on the bed (Figure 13-1).

A. _____

B. _____

C. _____

D. _____

E. _____

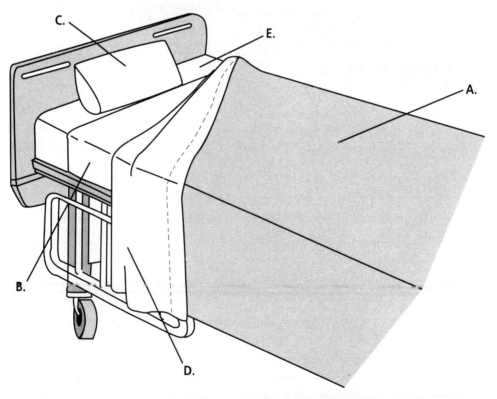

Figure 13-1

True or False

Directions: In the space provided, mark the statement "T" for true or "F" for false. If false, change the statement to make it true.

1. _____ Provide privacy for your client before making an occupied bed.
2. _____ Always wear gloves when handling linens stained with body fluids.
3. _____ The materials you use to make the bed depend on the client's needs and what is available.
4. _____ If the top sheet is not soiled, it may be reused as a bottom sheet.
5. _____ Use a dry cleaner's bag if the bed needs a plastic drawsheet.
6. _____ A closed bed is made while the client remains in the bed.
7. _____ When possible, get your client out of bed before making it.
8. _____ Roll soiled linens away from your clothing.
9. _____ Shake the bed linens to remove any crumbs.
10. _____ Do not place your client directly on a plastic drawsheet.
11. _____ Hold soiled linens close to you so you won't drop them on the floor.
12. _____ Fanfold the top bedding to the foot of the bed to open a closed bed.
13. _____ A bed cradle is used to lift top bedding off the client's feet.
14. _____ The most important reason for making a clean, neat, wrinkle-free bed is to look nice.
15. _____ Wash the egg crate foam mattress when it becomes soiled.

14

Personal Care

Procedures

Directions: Listed below are six procedures used to assist clients with personal care and grooming. For each procedure, review the steps listed and number them in the correct order.

1. Giving a back rub
   _____ Remove excess lotion with towel.
   _____ Place client on side or abdomen to expose entire back.
   _____ Remove clothing from upper body.
   _____ Rub hands together to warm lotion.
   _____ Use long, firm, but gentle strokes—up, out, and down.
   _____ Provide privacy (close door, shut drapes, pull shades).

2. Giving a complete bed bath
   _____ Wash the genital and rectal areas.
   _____ Give a back rub.
   _____ Remove soiled towels and washcloth and place in area to be washed.
   _____ Wash and dry leg while other foot is soaking.
   _____ Obtain materials.
   _____ Wash eye areas gently with clean water only.

3. Giving a shower in the bathtub
   _____ Adjust water temperature and water pressure.
   _____ Assist client into tub and to use grab bars.
   _____ Clean tub and remove towels to area to be washed.
   _____ Place nonskid mat in tub.
   _____ Place bath chair in tub.
   _____ Check temperature of bathroom for warmth and to see that it is free of drafts.

4. Shaving the male client using a blade razor

_____ Explain what you are going to do.

_____ Put on gloves.

_____ Wet and lather client's face.

_____ Remove gloves and wash your hands.

_____ Shave in direction of hair growth.

_____ Obtain materials.

5. Caring for client's hair

_____ Brush hair, section by section, from root to end of hair.

_____ Explain what you are going to do.

_____ Wash your hands.

_____ Place bath towel around client's shoulders.

_____ Remove towel.

_____ Arrange hair as client wishes.

6. Caring for dentures

_____ Assist client to remove dentures from mouth.

_____ Wash your hands and put on gloves.

_____ Fill sink with warm water.

_____ Assist client to replace dentures in mouth.

_____ Brush dentures with toothpaste and rinse.

_____ Obtain materials.

True or False

Directions: In the space provided, mark the statement "T" for true or "F" for false. If false, change the statement to make it true.

1. _____ All clients need complete personal care.
2. _____ Oral hygiene means care of mouth including teeth, gums, and tongue.
3. _____ Dentures are cleaned in hot, soapy water.
4. _____ Older adults may take a tub bath or shower twice a week.
5. _____ Not everyone needs a daily bath.
6. _____ Partial baths may be given in bed, at bedside, or in the bathroom.
7. _____ Any chair may be used in the shower.
8. _____ The proper water temperature for a bath or shower is 109° F (42.7° C).
9. _____ Electric razors are not used when clients are receiving oxygen because there is danger that an electrical spark could cause a fire.
10. _____ When helping clients to dress, put clothing on the weak side first.
11. _____ With range-of-motion (ROM) exercises, the client lifts weights and does deep knee bends.
12. _____ Stop ROM if you feel resistance or tightness in a joint.
13. _____ Do as much as you can for your client. This will help him/her get better faster.
14. _____ Always wear gloves when shaving a client's face with a blade razor.
15. _____ False teeth should be stored in a denture box or cup.

What Needs To Be Corrected?

Directions: In the figures that follow, there are problems with personal care. In the space provided, explain how you would correct the picture.

1. (Figure 14-1)
    A. What's wrong?

   _____

    B. Correction

   _____

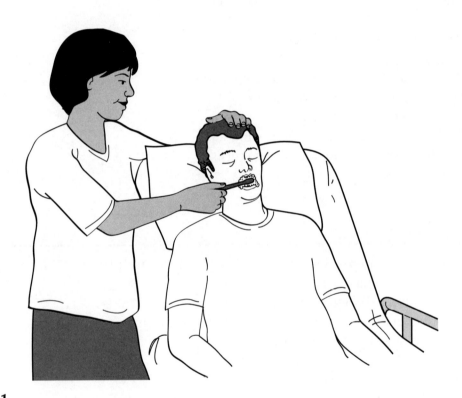

Figure 14-1

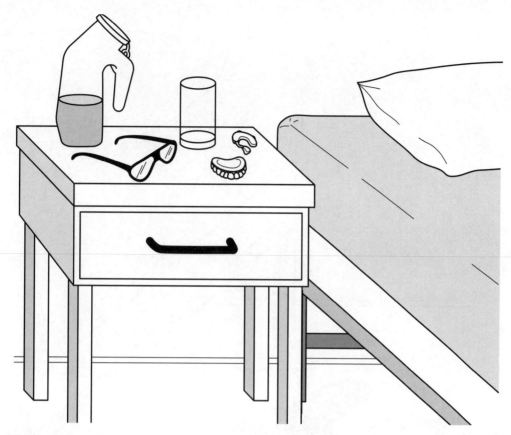

Figure 14-2

2. (Figure 14-2)
    A. What's wrong?

    _____

    B. Correction

    _____

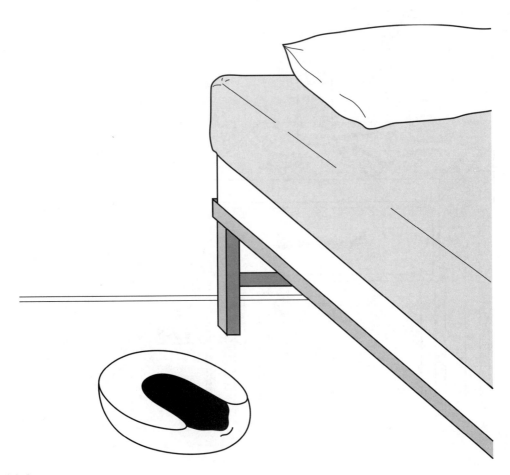

Figure 14-3

3. (Figure 14-3)
   A. What's wrong?

   _____

   B. Correction

   _____

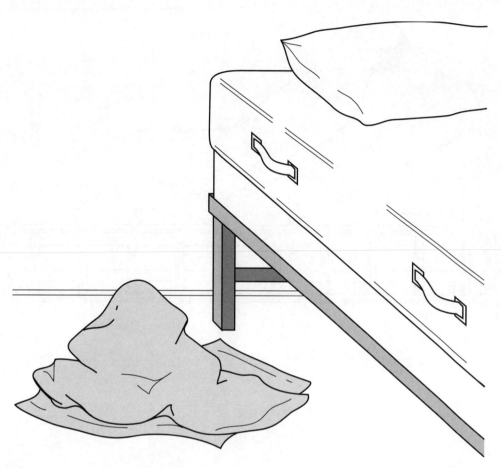

Figure 14-4

4. (Figure 14-4)
   A. What's wrong?

   _____

   B. Correction

   _____

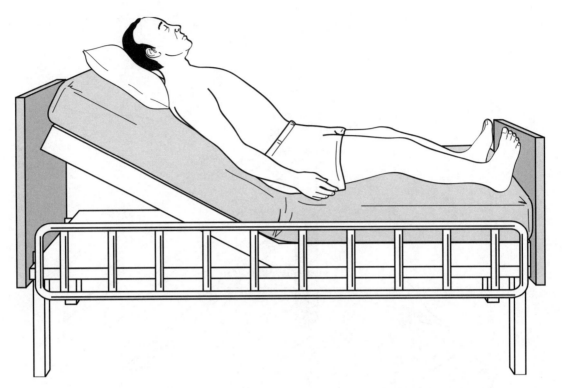

Figure 14-5

5. (Figure 14-5)
   A. What's wrong?

   _____

   B. Correction

   _____

15

Elimination

Procedures

Directions: Listed below are four procedures used to assist clients with elimination. For each procedure, review the steps listed and number them in the correct order.

1. Giving and removing a bedpan
   _____ Give toilet paper and ask client to call when finished.
   _____ Place client in flat position and remove bedpan.
   _____ Raise bed to convenient working height.
   _____ Cleanse perineal area with toilet tissue, if necessary, wiping from front to back.
   _____ Warm bedpan with warm tap water. Dry with paper towels.
   _____ Cover bedpan, take to bathroom, and empty contents.
2. Giving and removing a urinal
   _____ Give urinal to client so he can position it properly.
   _____ Help client to wash hands.
   _____ Rinse urinal with cold water; clean and disinfect.
   _____ Put on gloves and remove urinal.
   _____ Assist client to stand.
   _____ Put urinal away; remove and discard gloves.
3. Care of the client with an indwelling catheter
   _____ Record what you have done and report any abnormal conditions.
   _____ Put on gloves.
   _____ Tape and position catheter properly.
   _____ Give perineal care.
   _____ Remove plastic drawsheet or incontinence pad.
   _____ Wash catheter tube in a downward motion away from the urinary meatus for approximately 4 inches (20 cm).
4. Applying a condom catheter
   _____ Put on gloves.
   _____ Connect catheter tip to drainage tubing.
   _____ Give perineal care.

_____ Remove and discard gloves.

_____ If condom catheter is present, remove gently and place in plastic bag.

_____ Hold penis firmly and roll condom catheter onto penis with drainage opening at the urinary meatus.

What Needs To Be Corrected?

Directions: In the pictures below, there are problems with catheter bags and tubing. In the space provided, write what is wrong with the picture and how you will correct it.

1. (Figure 15-1)

   A. What's wrong?

   _____

   B. Correction

   _____

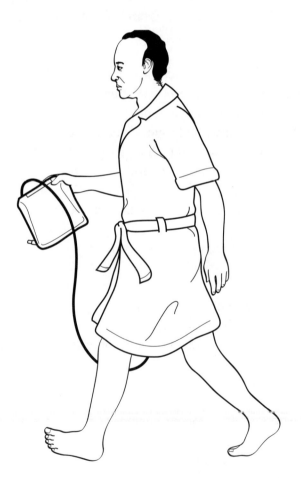

Figure 15-1

2. (Figure 15-2)
   A. What's wrong?

   B. Correction

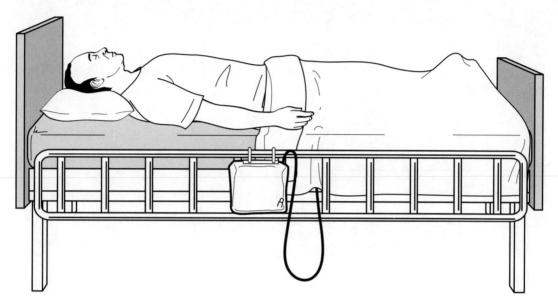

Figure 15-2

3. (Figure 15-3)
   A. What's wrong?

   B. Correction

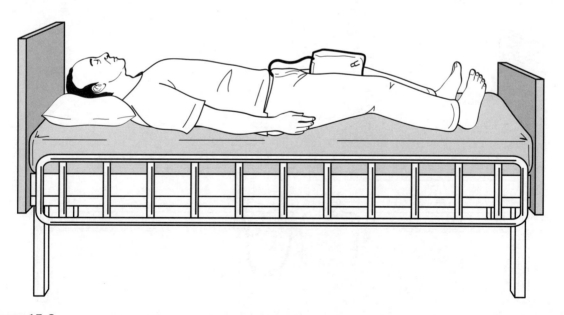

Figure 15-3

4. (Figure 15-4)
   A. What's wrong?

   _____

   B. Correction

   _____

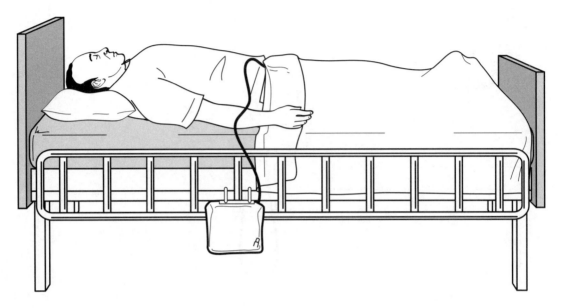

Figure 15-4

5. (Figure 15-5)
   A. What's wrong?

   _____

   B. Correction

   _____

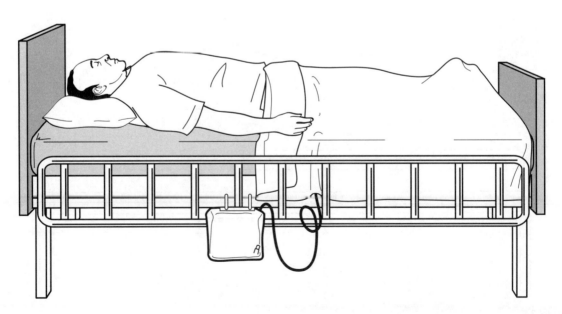

Figure 15-5

Situations

Directions: In the space provided, answer the questions for each situation.

1. Your client is on I&O. During the 4 hours that you provide care for Mr. Abud, he:

   Voids 375 ml of urine

   Drinks one cup of tea

   Eats two 8-oz cups of gelatin and four crackers

   Has one small bowel movement.

   At the end of the 4 hours, you record the I&O as follows:

   I = _____ ml

   O = _____ ml and _____.

2. Miss O'Brien was in the hospital for 3 weeks. During that time, she had difficulty with bowel elimination. Now that she is home, the doctor wants her to reestablish her normal bowel habits. Miss O'Brien uses the commode at her bedside. List three things you can do to help her regain regular bowel habits.

   _____

   _____

   _____

3. Your client, Juanita, has an indwelling catheter. While giving her perineal care, you observe that the area around the catheter is leaking urine and the skin is very reddened. She says the area is painful and she always has the feeling of wanting to use the commode. List two actions that you would take to handle this situation.

   _____

   _____

   _____

4. Mr. Patel has a colostomy. He is learning to care for it himself but needs help with unclamping and draining the pouch of fecal material. His companion tells you that he cries a lot after the registered nurse visits to instruct him about caring for the colostomy.

   A. What will you say to the companion?

   _____

   _____

   B. List three duties you may need to perform when helping Mr. Patel with colostomy care.

   _____

   _____

   _____

Completion

Directions: Fill in the missing word(s) on the blank line(s) for each statement.

1. Three characteristics of normal urine are _____, _____, and _____.
2. Two characteristics of a normal bowel movement (BM) are _____ and _____.
3. The medical term to describe air or gas in the intestine that is passed through the rectum is _____.
4. Two kinds of gas-forming foods are _____ and _____.
5. When clients are not able to control urination and/or bowel movements, the medical term to use is _____.
6. If you notice changes in your client's urine or bowel movements, notify _____ _____.
7. Your client has not had a BM for over 1 week and complains of abdominal discomfort. Also, you notice that small amounts of fecal liquid leak out of the anus. These may be signs that your client has a _____.
8. Waste materials are eliminated from the body by _____, _____, _____, and _____.
9. The medical term for material eliminated from the large intestine is _____.
10. The medical term to describe the process of eliminating solid waste through the anus is _____.
11. When waste products in the large intestine move so rapidly that water is not able to be absorbed, the term used is _____.
12. When providing perineal care or removing a bedpan, it is important to _____.
13. Three ways to help clients to maintain normal urination are:
    A. _____
    B. _____
    C. _____

16

Collecting Specimens

Procedures

Directions: Listed below are three procedures used to collect clients' specimens. For each procedure, review the steps listed and number them in the correct order.

1. Collecting a routine urine specimen
   _____ Pour urine into graduate and then into specimen container until 3/4 full.
   _____ Label container.
   _____ Store specimen in refrigerator.
   _____ Have client void into commode, bedpan, urinal, or "hat."
   _____ Put lid on specimen container.
   _____ Remove and discard gloves.

2. Collecting a stool specimen
   _____ Explain what you are going to do.
   _____ Transfer stool to specimen container using tongue depressor.
   _____ Label container.
   _____ Put on gloves.
   _____ Record what you have done and report any abnormal conditions to your supervisor.
   _____ Flush remaining feces down toilet and assist client to complete toileting, as necessary.

3. Collecting a sputum specimen
   _____ Place container into plastic bag, then into paper bag.
   _____ Have client hold sputum specimen container.
   _____ Remove and discard gloves.
   _____ Obtain materials.
   _____ Do not touch the inside of the container. Keep the outside clean and free of any sputum.
   _____ Assist client to rinse mouth with plain water.

True or False

Directions: In the space provided, mark the statement "T" for true or "F" for false. If false, change the statement to make it true.

1. _____ Specimens are small amounts of body tissue or fluids that are collected for examination and analysis in the medical laboratory.
2. _____ Have client discard used lancets directly into the garbage can.
3. _____ Label specimen container as follows: client's name and agency's name.
4. _____ Specimen containers are capped tightly to avoid contamination from spilling.
5. _____ All specimens should be double bagged—in a plastic bag or wrap and then in a paper bag.
6. _____ It is usually easier for the client to expel sputum for a specimen in the early morning after arising.
7. _____ Completely fill the urine specimen container in order to have enough urine for examination.
8. _____ Wear gloves when collecting specimens only when you think you may spill them.
9. _____ Collect 5 oz of stool for a specimen.
10. _____ When collecting a 24-hour urine specimen starting at 3 PM, Thursday, place the first specimen voided at 3 PM and the specimen voided at 3 PM on Friday into the container.

Crossword Puzzle

Directions: Complete the crossword puzzle by identifying important terms found in Chapter 16.

ACROSS

2. Type of urine specimen
4. Semi-solid waste from the large intestine
7. Specimens are sent here
9. Produced by the kidneys
10. Short, pointed blades
11. Organisms that live in or on another organism

DOWN

1. Determining the substances present in a specimen
3. Dirty, containing pathogens
5. Specimen is placed in this object
6. Worn when handling specimens
8. Stones formed in the body

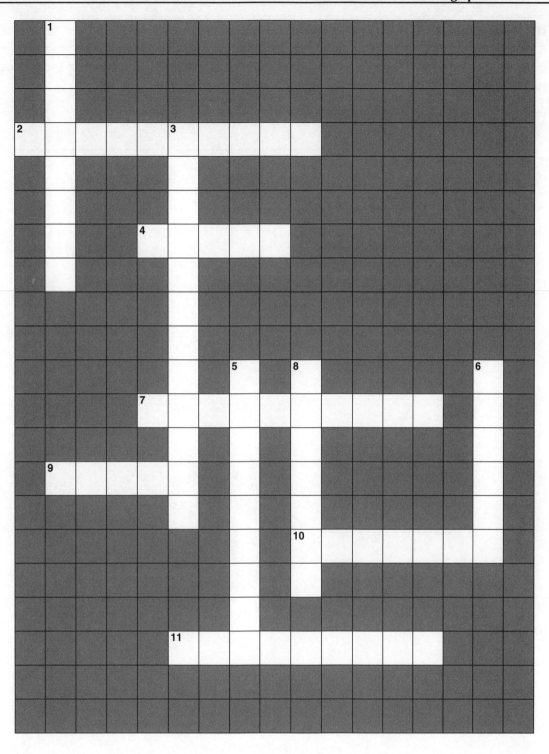

What Needs To Be Corrected?

Directions: In the pictures below, there are problems with specimen collection. In the space provided, write what is wrong with the picture and how you will correct it.

1. (Figure 16-1)

    A. What's wrong?

    _____

    B. Correction

    _____

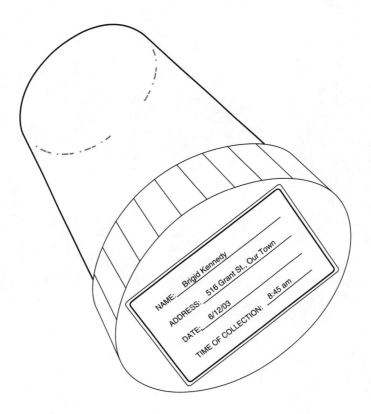

NAME: _____ Brigid Kennedy _____

ADDRESS: _____ 516 Grant St., Our Town _____

DATE: _____ 6/12/03 _____

TIME OF COLLECTION: _____ 8:45 am _____

Figure 16-1

2. (Figure 16-2)
   A. What's wrong?

   _____

   B. Correction

   _____

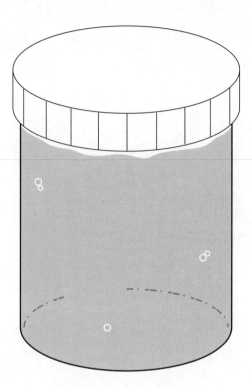

Figure 16-2

3. (Figure 16-3)
   A. What's wrong?

   _____

   B. Correction

   _____

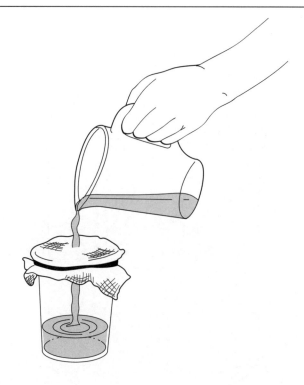

Figure 16-3

4. (Figure 16-4)
   A. What's wrong?

   _____

   B. Correction

   _____

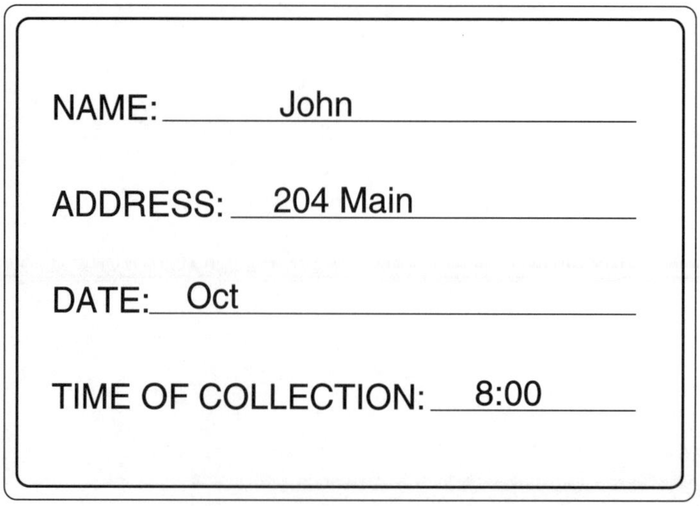

NAME: _____John_____

ADDRESS: ___204 Main_____

DATE: __Oct_____

TIME OF COLLECTION: ___8:00_____

Figure 16-4

17

Measuring Vital Signs

Reading the Thermometer

Directions: Below are drawings of thermometers (Figures 17-1 *A* through *F*). Read each thermometer and place the reading in the space provided.

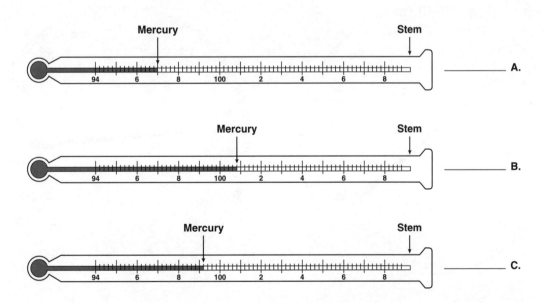

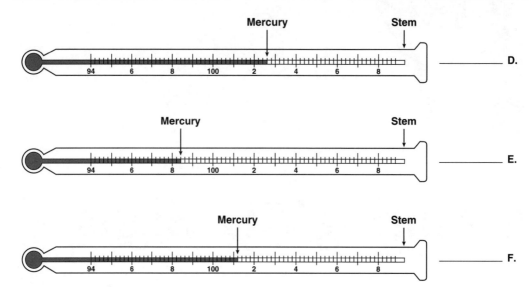

Figure 17-1

Reading the Dial of the Blood Pressure Cuff

Directions: Below are drawings of dials. Read each dial's indicator and place the reading in the space provided (Figures 17-2 *A* through *D*).

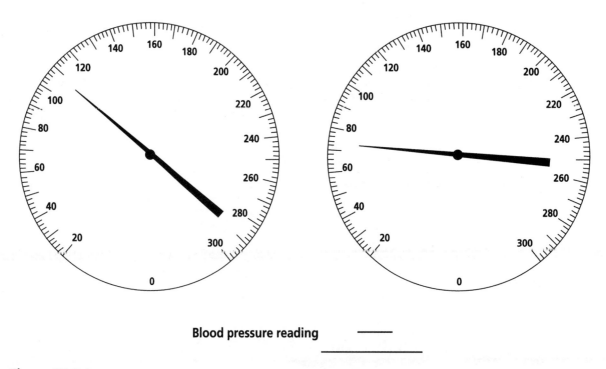

Blood pressure reading _____

Figure 17-2 A

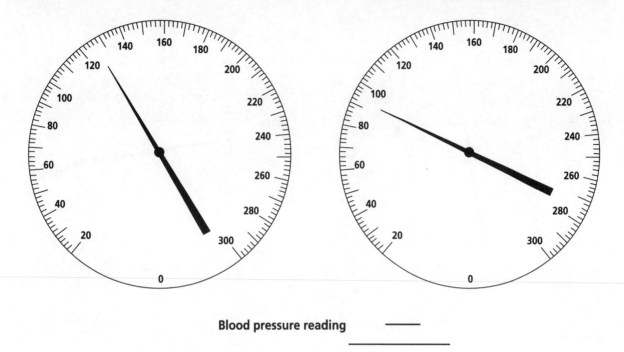

Blood pressure reading ———

_____

Figure 17-2 B

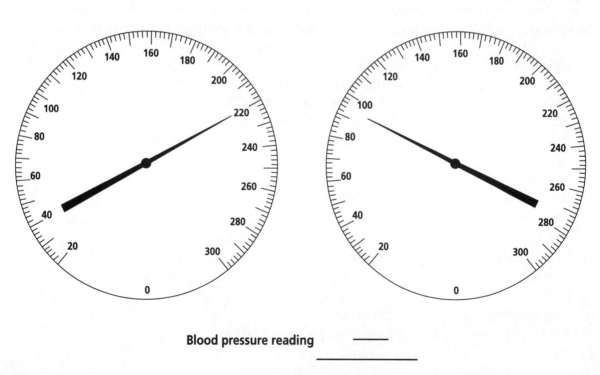

Blood pressure reading ———

_____

Figure 17-2 C

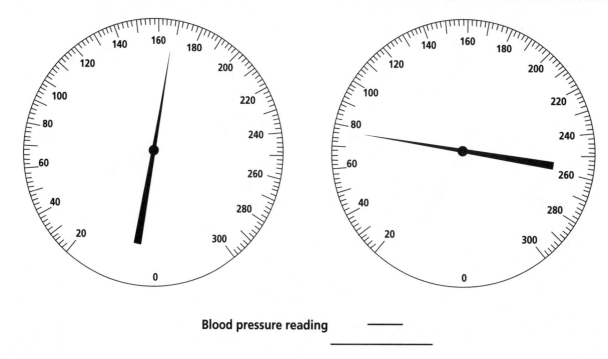

Blood pressure reading ———

Figure 17-2 D

Matching

Directions: Match the terms in Column A with the correct definition in Column B.

COLUMN A
A. Chestpiece
B. Axillary
C. Inhalation
D. Radial artery
E. Systole
F. Stethoscope
G. Exhalation
H. Blood pressure
I. Diastole
J. Thermometer
K. Brachial artery
L. Dial
M. Hypertension
N. Vital signs
O. Pulse rate

COLUMN B
1. ____ measures body heat
2. ____ high blood pressure
3. ____ blood vessel used to measure BP
4. ____ part of blood pressure cuff that shows numbers from 20 to 300 and has a pointer
5. ____ resting part of heart beat
6. ____ part of stethoscope
7. ____ temperature, pulse, respirations, and blood pressure
8. ____ contracting part of heart beat
9. ____ removing carbon dioxide
10. ____ instrument used to hear sounds in the body
11. ____ number of heart beats in 1 minute
12. ____ in the armpit
13. ____ located on palm side of the wrist at base of thumb
14. ____ measurement of force of blood against wall of an artery
15. ____ breathing in oxygen

Reporting Vital Signs

Directions: Listed below are recordings of vital signs. Review this list and, in the space provided, place an "X" beside the ones you would report to your supervisor.

1. ____ T. 103.2° F (O) (39.5° C)
2. ____ P. 72, regular
3. ____ T. 98.6° F (O) (37° C)
4. ____ R. 10 with wheezing and pain
5. ____ P. 123, weak
6. ____ T. 99.5° F (T) (37.5° C)
7. ____ BP $\frac{118}{70}$
8. ____ BP $\frac{220}{94}$
9. ____ BP $\frac{70}{30}$
10. ____ R. 16, periods of no breathing, then rapid breathing
11. ____ T. 99.6° F (O) (37.5° C)
12. ____ P. 69, irregular
13. ____ T. 96.8° F (A) (36° C)
14. ____ T. 100.6° F (R) (38.1° C)
15. ____ T. 102.2° F (O) (39° C)

Completion

Directions: Fill in the missing word(s) on the blank line(s) for each statement.

1. Vital signs give important information about the body processes of _____, _____, and _____.
2. Take the client's vital signs when the client is _____.
3. Factors that cause vital signs to increase are _____, _____, and _____.
4. Heat leaves the body by means of _____ and _____.
5. It is 9:30 AM. Your client has just had a big cup of hot coffee. Take the oral temperature at _____.
6. Have the client hold the glass thermometer in the mouth for _____ minutes before you remove and read the thermometer.
7. To read the glass thermometer, hold it at _____ level.
8. Remove the electronic thermometer and read the digital display window when you hear the _____.
9. Read the _____ dot to change color on the disposable thermometer.
10. Your client has diarrhea. Do not take a _____ temperature.
11. The "normal" systolic pressure in an adult is _____. The "normal" diastolic pressure in an adult is _____.

12. The normal range of TPRs in adults is:

    T (O) _____

    P   _____

    R   _____

13. Before and after using the stethoscope, clean earpieces and chestpiece to prevent _____ of _____.

14. Shake down the oral glass thermometer to _____ before placing it under the client's tongue.

15. When cleaning the rectal thermometer, begin at the _____ and wipe _____ toward the _____. Use a _____ motion.

16. Do not use your _____ to take your client's pulse.

17. You begin to take your client's pulse at 10:35 AM. You finish taking this pulse at _____ AM. You continue holding the pulse while you take the respirations. You finish taking the respirations at _____ AM.

18

Special Procedures

Situations

Directions: Listed below are four situations you may experience as a home care aide. Read each situation and answer the questions in the spaces provided.

1. Olga has a chronic respiratory disease. She has difficulty breathing and receives oxygen by nasal cannula. While giving her a bed bath, you notice that the skin above her ears and around her nostrils is reddened where the plastic tubing comes in contact with these areas. Olga's lips are chapped and she complains that her mouth is always dry.
   A. List at least three activities that you can perform to make Olga more comfortable.

   _____

   _____

   _____

   _____

   _____

   B. As a home care aide, you know that oxygen is one of the three ingredients needed for a fire. List five safety precautions to take when Olga is receiving oxygen.

   _____

   _____

   _____

   _____

   _____

2. You have been caring for Moishe, a man aged 79 years with diabetes, for several months. In addition to light housekeeping duties, the care plan indicates the following:
   • Apply clean, dry dressing to the reddened area of the lower left leg daily
   • Warm soaks to left foot for 20 minutes daily
   A. List four signs you will watch for when applying the warm soaks.

   _____

   _____

   _____

   _____

B. How frequently will you check for these signs and why?

_____

_____

_____

_____

C. When removing the tape on the dressing, you notice that the skin is very red. You also notice that there is a small amount of greenish drainage on the dressing. List two actions you will take.

_____

_____

3. Emmie Lou has severe arthritis. She lives with her daughter and three grandchildren, who are all under the age of 5 years. During the past two visits, her daughter has complained about the time it takes for her to care for her mother, including giving the vitamin B_{12} injection. "If only her hands and eyesight were better, Mama could take care of herself and give herself the shot, too. These kids take a lot of my time." Today, as you finish giving Emmie Lou a shower, her daughter says, "Let me teach you how to give the vitamin shot. It's really very easy to do. You know how much Mama and I trust you. Besides, vitamins are not drugs, so you can give them. If I can do it, you certainly can do it even better."

A. What is your response to the daughter?

_____

_____

_____

_____

_____

B. What will you do?

_____

_____

_____

_____

4. Your client, Mrs. Choi, has problems with her heart and circulation, especially in her legs. The care plan indicates that you are to assist her in taking her heart medication and help her to put on the elastic stockings after the bed bath. Mrs. Choi is usually not a complainer, but today she tells you about the severe cramps she had in her legs during the night. "I didn't want to wake up my husband—he needs his sleep. Please don't tell anyone about this, I'm sure they'll go away."

A. What is your response to Mrs. Choi?

_____

_____

_____

_____

B. What will you do?

_____

_____

_____

_____

C. When you remove the cap on the medication bottle, you notice that the pills are discolored and are crumbling. What two actions will you take?

_____

_____

_____

_____

Procedures

Directions: Listed below are three special procedures that may be performed by the home care aide. For each procedure, review the steps listed and number them in the correct order.

1. Giving a sitz bath
_____ Ask client to void.
_____ Place sitz bowl so that drainage holes are at the back of the toilet.
_____ Ask client to remove and discard dressing or pad, if worn. Assist, if needed.
_____ Fill half of plastic sitz bowl with warm water, 94° to 98° F (34° to 37° C).
_____ Dry area and reapply dressing or pad, if necessary.
_____ Instruct client to open clamp of water bag to let warmer water into bowl.

2. Applying hot compresses
_____ Wring out compress and apply to area.
_____ Fill basin or container $\frac{1}{2}$ to $\frac{2}{3}$ full of water at 105° to 115° F (40.5° to 46.1° C).
_____ Check client's skin every 10 minutes for danger signs.
_____ Cover compress quickly with plastic wrap.
_____ Place waterproof protector pad under the body part where compress is to be applied.
_____ Put on gloves.

3. Applying elastic stocking
_____ Place foot of stocking over client's toes, foot, and heel.
_____ Put client in supine position.
_____ Record what you have done.
_____ Adjust stocking to fit smoothly without folds or wrinkles.
_____ Turn stocking inside out, down to the heel.
_____ Fit client's foot into heel and toe portion of stocking.

4. Assisting with transdermal disks
_____ Have client remove and discard old disk into waste container.
_____ Record what you have done.
_____ Observe as client applies new disk to skin surface.
_____ Ask client to select site for new disk.
_____ Wash skin that had been covered by old disk.
_____ Obtain materials.

Matching

Directions: Match the terms listed in Column B with the correct definition in Column A.

COLUMN A

_____ 1. Medications that can be bought without a prescription

_____ 2. Gas needed by all cells in the body

_____ 3. Small gelatin container that holds medication

_____ 4. Inside a vein

_____ 5. Absorbed through the skin

_____ 6. A two-pronged device that delivers oxygen; short prongs are inserted into client's nostrils

_____ 7. Solid forms of medication for insertion into a body cavity

_____ 8. A blood clot

_____ 9. Small cylinders containing a drug that is inhaled in specifically measured (metered) doses

_____ 10. A blood clot that travels through the circulatory system until it lodges in a distant blood vessel

COLUMN B

A. Capsule

B. Transdermal

C. Suppositories

D. Metered dose inhaler (MDI)

E. Intravenous

F. OTC

G. Oxygen

H. Nasal cannula

I. Thrombus

J. Embolus

True or False

Directions: In the space provided, mark the statement "T" for true or "F" for false. If false, change the statement to make it true.

1. _____ Medications are substances used in the treatment of disease or illness.

2. _____ Over-the-counter drugs can be purchased without a prescription.

3. _____ Oral medications should be taken with a small sip of water.

4. _____ Clients place sublingual tablets under the tongue.

5. _____ Topical medications and transdermal disks are both applied to the skin.

6. _____ The method in which medication is taken is called the route.

7. _____ The amount of medication to be taken is called the dose.

8. _____ When one dose is forgotten or omitted, it's OK for the client to take a double dose the next time.

9. _____ If your client says the tablets are the wrong shape and color, tell him/her to take them anyway.

10. _____ If your client does not take a medication, notify your supervisor.

11. _____ Record if a medication is not taken (or omitted) and why.

12. _____ Unused medications should be saved, because they might be needed again.

13. _____ Vaseline may be used to lubricate a rectal suppository.

14. _____ Transdermal disks are usually applied to the chest or upper arm.

15. _____ Older adults are at great risk for burns from applications of heat.

16. _____ When applying heat or cold, be sure to check the client's skin every 30 minutes.

17. _____ Hot compresses are an example of moist heat.

18. _____ Sitz baths may be given by having the client soak in the bathtub.

19. _____ Oxygen is a drug and is part of the client's treatment or therapy.

20. _____ "No Smoking" and "Oxygen in Use" signs are placed on the front door of the residence where oxygen is being used.
21. _____ Home care aides may regulate the flow of intravenous fluids.
22. _____ A blood clot is called a thrombus.
23. _____ Elastic stockings should be removed three times a day to check the color and warmth of the client's legs and feet.
24. _____ Improper application of elastic stockings or elastic bandages can block circulation and cause damage to tissues.
25. _____ Elastic bandages should be applied as tightly as possible.

What Needs To Be Corrected?

Directions: In the following figures there are problems with special procedures. In the space provided, explain how you would correct the picture.

1. (Figure 18-1)

_____

_____

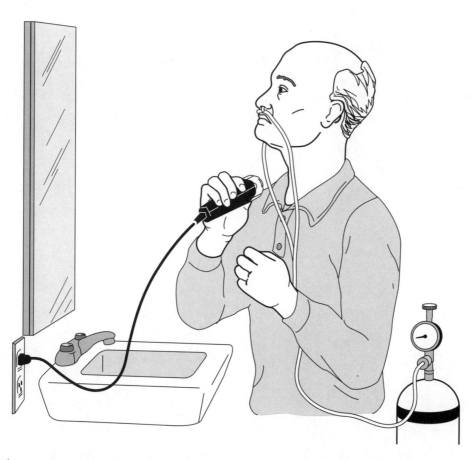

Figure 18-1

2. (Figure 18-2)

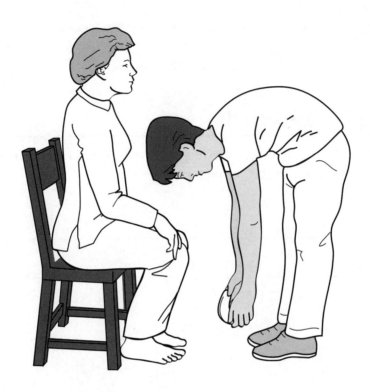

Figure 18-2

3. (Figure 18-3)

_____

_____

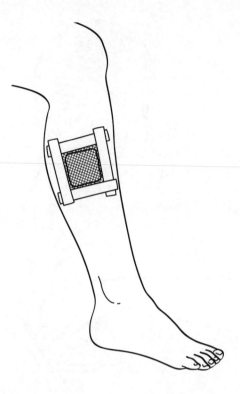

Figure 18-3

4. (Figure 18-4)

_____

_____

_____

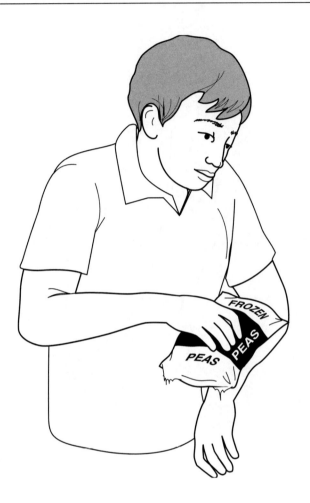

Figure 18-4

19

Caring for Older Adults

True or False

Directions: In the space provided, mark the statement "T" for true or "F" for false. If false, change the statement to make it true.

1. _____ Aging begins at age 65 years.
2. _____ Incontinence is normal for clients who are older than 80 years.
3. _____ There are more older women than older men.
4. _____ As normal aging progresses, the older person's personality will surely change.
5. _____ Mental confusion is a normal part of growing old.
6. _____ Try to change the subject when your client begins to talk about the "old times."
7. _____ The need for home care will decrease in the future because the life span of older adults is decreasing.
8. _____ There are three categories of older adults—the young old, middle old, and oldest old.
9. _____ The rate at which we age depends on one factor only—our heredity.
10. _____ Loneliness is a common experience for many older adults.
11. _____ Older adults can't learn new things.
12. _____ Accepting oneself as an aging person is one of the adjustments older adults need to make.
13. _____ The population that is increasing at the most rapid rate is the 65 to 75 age-group.
14. _____ You do not need to explain what you are going to do for the older adult. He or she won't understand what you are saying.
15. _____ Twenty percent of older adults are cared for in institutions.

Normal Conditions of Aging

Directions: Below each of the normal conditions of aging listed, describe a way you can help your client to cope with the condition.

1. Difficulty adjusting to a dark room

   _____

   _____

2. Forgets where eyeglasses were placed

   _____

   _____

3. Dry skin

   _____

   _____

4. Dry mouth

   _____

   _____

5. Complains of being cold

   _____

   _____

6. Occasional constipation

   _____

   _____

7. Shortness of breath with increased activity

   _____

   _____

8. Anxious about changes in routine

   _____

   _____

9. Urgent need to void

   _____

   _____

10. Feeling bloated

    _____

    _____

11. Rapid heart beat when under stress

    _____

    _____

12. Trouble adjusting to depths (going up and down stairs)

    _____

    _____

13. Trouble understanding what you are saying

    _____

    _____

14. Thick, hard toenails

_____

_____

15. Unsteady balance when rising suddenly from a chair

_____

_____

Situations

Directions: Read each situation. Answer the questions in the space provided.

1. Mrs. Edwards, aged 75 years, has recently returned from the rehabilitation center where she learned to walk following a fractured hip. Today, her daughter, who is visiting for the day, greets you at the door and asks you to come into the kitchen. You can smell the odor of stale beer in the apartment. She closes the door and whispers, "I'm really worried about Mom. She's always liked a few beers while watching television at night but now she's drinking a six pack a day or more. Lately, she refuses to eat any meals. She just sits and drinks that beer and eats pretzels. Mom says that it's none of my business. Will you tell her not to drink? She won't listen to me." Later, while cleaning Mrs. Edwards' room, you notice that there are three cases of beer under the bed.

   A. How will you answer the daughter's question?

   _____

   _____

   _____

   _____

   _____

   B. What will you do with the three cases of beer?

   _____

   _____

   _____

   _____

   _____

   C. What will you do?

   _____

   _____

   _____

   _____

   _____

2. Magdalena is a frail woman aged 80 years who speaks very little English. She lives with her nephew and his wife. This is your first visit. The care plan indicates that you are to help Magdalena to take a shower, dress, walk, and change the bed linens. Her nephew greets you at the door and appears very upset. He says, "Last week, Auntie peed on the new sofa in the living room. Now, it's all ruined. She's never done anything like this before. We know that she did it on purpose, just to get even with us for not taking her to visit her grandson." He continued, "My wife is so angry that she locks her in the bedroom so that she won't ruin the rest of the furniture!" As he unlocks the bedroom door, you can hear Magdalena crying in bed. She speaks to you in Spanish. You do not understand what she is saying, but you know that she is terribly upset. The bed linens are dirty with urine and feces and it appears that the linens have not been changed for several days.

A. How will you respond to Magdalena?

B. What will you do?

C. What will you record?

D. What will you say to Magdalena's nephew?

3. Mr. Lewis, aged 79 years, has lived alone since his wife died 3 years ago. Recently, he was hospitalized for a heart condition. You have been caring for him three times a week for the past 2 weeks. Today, you notice that he is confused and dressed in dirty pajamas. In the kitchen, there is a stack of dirty dishes in the sink. On the table is the uneaten meal left by the Meals on Wheels volunteer yesterday.

What would you do? List four activities.

A.
B.
C.
D.

20

Caring for Mothers, Infants, and Children

Matching

Directions: Match the terms listed in Column B with the correct definition in Column A.

COLUMN A

_____ 1. Space covered by tough membranes between bones of infant's skull

_____ 2. Discharge from the vagina after childbirth

_____ 3. Colored, circular area surrounding the nipple

_____ 4. Educated guess about the probable outcome of an illness

_____ 5. First 6 weeks following the birth of the baby

_____ 6. System of rules that governs the way we act

_____ 7. Emotional attachment between infant and parents, especially the mother

_____ 8. The completion of the full 9 months of pregnancy

_____ 9. Normal reactions infants have that makes them begin to suck when their cheeks are stroked

_____ 10. Varicose veins in the rectum or anus

COLUMN B

A. Bond

B. Hemorrhoids

C. Fontanel

D. Discipline

E. Lochia

F. Full term

G. Prognosis

H. Rooting reflex

I. Areola

J. Postpartum period

Recognizing Normal and Abnormal Conditions in the Mother

Directions: Review the following list of observations. Place an "X" beside those conditions you would immediately report to your supervisor.

1. _____ Complains of discomfort in the perineal area

2. _____ Weight loss of 19 lbs (8.6 kg) on the 10th day following delivery

3. _____ Three pads are used within 1 hour and contain a large number of blood clots

4. _____ Hemorrhoids in the anal area

91

5. ____ Cracked skin around the left nipple

6. ____ Elevated temperature—101° F (38.4° C) or higher

7. ____ Complains of tenderness in calf muscle of right leg

8. ____ Brownish lochia on the ninth day following delivery

9. ____ Mother says, "I feel so sad today, I just want to cry."

10. ____ Breasts are painful and hot to the touch

11. ____ Refuses to drink fluids because "My breasts will dry up faster."

12. ____ Vaginal discharge has a foul odor

13. ____ Lochia is scant and cream-colored on the 20th day following delivery

14. ____ Mother eats only skim milk, gelatin, and dry crackers because she says, "I want to lose all the weight I gained. I hate being fat!"

15. ____ Tender breasts on the third day following delivery

16. ____ No bowel movements for 5 days

17. ____ Not interested in surroundings, withdrawn, and refuses to eat

18. ____ Swelling and redness around the abdominal incision (cesarean birth)

19. ____ Complains of being exhausted on the second and third days following delivery

20. ____ Worries about being able to care for the infant properly

Situations

Directions: In the space provided, answer the questions for each situation.

1. You are scheduled to visit Amanda, who is a single mother aged 17 years. Her baby, Jeffrey, is now 8 days old. Both mother and baby are well and healthy. The professional nurse has been visiting Amanda to help her learn how to care for Jeffrey.

   Today, you find Amanda lying on her bed and sobbing. Between sobs, she tells you, "I'll never learn to be a good mother. The baby cries all the time; I can't get him to breast-feed right away; I worry that the pins will hurt him when I change his diapers. I never thought being a mother would be such hard work! Where is my boyfriend to help me?"

   A. How will you communicate with Amanda?

   _____
   _____
   _____
   _____
   _____

   B. What will you do?

   _____
   _____
   _____
   _____
   _____

2. Just after Yolanda Potts brought her new baby home from the hospital, her older child, Johnny, says, "I don't like that baby. She stinks!" Johnny is 4 years of age and has been toilet trained for a year but now becomes incontinent. Yolanda tells the home care aide, "I am so tired with a new baby. Johnny is acting like a baby, too. I could just smack him."

List three things you would do.

A. _____
   _____

B. _____
   _____

C. _____
   _____

True or False

Directions: In the space provided, mark the statement "T" for true or "F" for false. If false, change the statement to make it true.

1. ____ An infant is given a tub bath after the umbilical stump falls off.
2. ____ Newborn infants are awake most of the day.
3. ____ Sleeping infants should be placed on their backs.
4. ____ The stool of a breast-fed infant is dark brown and formed.
5. ____ Infants are burped only at the end of every feeding.
6. ____ The first breast "milk" is known as colostrum.
7. ____ Infants chill quickly, and their hands and feet become bluish and cold.
8. ____ The umbilical stump falls off after 2 weeks.
9. ____ Newborn infants eat four times a day.
10. ____ Bottles of formula may be warmed in the microwave.
11. ____ Test the temperature of baby bath water on your elbow.
12. ____ Mothers should be in a comfortable position when they are breast or bottle feeding.
13. ____ Children do not react to stress.
14. ____ Follow (client's) family rules regarding discipline.
15. ____ Children often use nonverbal communication as a means of expressing emotional response to stress.

Observation

Directions: Review the following list of observations of a normal newborn infant. Place an "X" beside those conditions you would immediately report to your supervisor.

1. ____ yellow skin
2. ____ bluish and cold hands and feet
3. ____ spitting up small amounts of feeding when burped
4. ____ crying and fussing every 3 hours
5. ____ wet diaper at every feeding
6. ____ sleeping most of the time
7. ____ crying constantly; cannot be comforted
8. ____ limp, hardly moves or cries
9. ____ has several yellow bowel movements a day
10. ____ cries during bath

Caring for Clients With Mental Illness

Crossword Puzzle

Directions: Complete the crossword puzzle by identifying important terms found in Chapter 21.

ACROSS

2. Use of violent or abusive behavior to cope with anxiety
3. A sudden uncontrollable urge
4. Feeling of being extremely frightened and unable to move
8. Fearful about real or imagined threats to a person's well-being
9. Returning to behavior, thought, or feelings used at an earlier stage of development
10. False beliefs held as true, in spite of evidence to the contrary

DOWN

1. Term used to describe the misuse of chemical substances that leads to an emotional or physical dependence
5. Mental state in which a client is disoriented about time, place, or person
6. A disorder characterized by feelings of extreme sadness and hopelessness
7. Sensory perception (things seen, heard, felt, and smelled) that aren't actually there

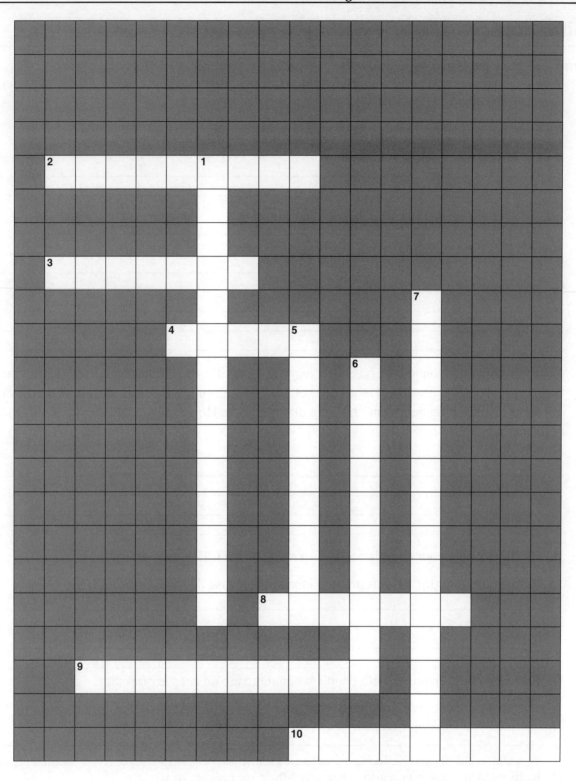

Situations

Directions: In the space provided, answer the questions for each situation.

1. Your client is overactive, constantly pacing back and forth throughout the home. How will you meet her needs that are listed below?

   A. Food and fluids

   B. Elimination

   C. Hygiene and grooming

2. George's wife tells you that he has been very confused. He tries to put on his socks after putting on his shoes; begins to get ready for bed at 9 A.M., thinking that it is evening; and tries to drink the dishwashing detergent, thinking that it is soda. How can you help George with each of these problems?

3. How will you meet your client's needs, as a result of the following behaviors:

   A. Refuses to eat or drink fluids prepared for him because they are "poison."

   B. Carries on conversations with people when there are no people present.

   C. Refuses to take the medications because "they are poison, too."

4. Your client is depressed and sad most of the day. He cries easily and tells you, "I'm too tired to even lift a fork or glass to feed myself." He also tells you that he doesn't even have the energy to go to the bathroom.

   How would you meet his need for:

   A. Foods and fluids

   _____
   _____
   _____

   B. Elimination

   _____
   _____
   _____

   He says, "I can't stand feeling like this anymore—maybe I should just end it all."

   C. What should you say?

   _____
   _____
   _____
   _____
   _____

   D. What should you do?

   _____
   _____
   _____
   _____
   _____

5. Your elderly client is very confused. She sometimes gets out of the house, stands on the front porch, and takes off all of her clothes. Other times she removes her clothing and stands by the window exposing herself.

   A. What measures may prevent this behavior?

   _____
   _____
   _____
   _____

   B. What can you do if this does happen?

   _____
   _____
   _____
   _____
   _____

6. Your client is recovering from injuries received in an automobile accident. He uses a wheel-chair to get about his apartment and needs assistance with ADL, especially hygiene and grooming. When you reach into the top drawer of his bureau to get his electric razor, you discover several small cellophane bags containing a white powder and a syringe.

   A. What should you do?

   _____

   _____

   _____

   _____

7. Your client's daughter says, "I can't stand my mother since she got sick and I have to take care of her. The only thing that helps is this." She lights a marijuana cigarette. She invites you to join her, saying, "Have some, dearie, it'll make life a lot easier."

   A. What should you say?

   _____

   _____

   _____

   _____

   B. What should you do?

   _____

   _____

   _____

   _____

22

Caring for Clients With Illnesses Requiring Home Care

Client Conditions

Directions: You are caring for eight clients during the week. Each client has one of the following conditions. Below each condition, describe two activities you will perform to assist your client.

1. Wandering

_____
_____
_____
_____

2. Fatigue

_____
_____
_____
_____

3. Difficulty swallowing

_____
_____
_____
_____

4. Pain

_____
_____
_____
_____

5. Paralysis or weakness on right side of the body

_____
_____
_____
_____

6. Diarrhea

_____
_____
_____
_____

7. Difficulty breathing

_____
_____
_____
_____

8. Sores in the mouth

_____
_____
_____
_____

Situations

1. Mrs. Gable's daughter was worried about her mother for more than a year. She noticed that her mother became more forgetful and confused. Her personality seemed to change, too. These were real concerns, especially because Mrs. Gable lived alone. One evening, as her daughter entered the front door of Mrs. Gable's home, she smelled something burning. In the kitchen, her mother had placed a frozen dinner, carton and all, into a frying pan and turned on the stove. She arrived just in time to put out the fire. The next week, the daughter took her mother to the doctor for a check-up. After further testing, Mrs. Gable was diagnosed as having Alzheimer's disease. Now, Mrs. Gable lives with her daughter. You live next to the daughter.

   A. The daughter asks your advice about making her home safer for her mother. List five suggestions you will give her.
      1. _____
      2. _____
      3. _____
      4. _____
      5. _____

   B. Mrs. Gable hides her eyeglasses, then she can't find them. How will you advise the daughter about how to handle this situation?

      _____
      _____
      _____
      _____

C. Mrs. Gable cannot remember the names of her daughter, son-in-law, and two grandchildren. This makes her very upset. What will you suggest to help remember their names?

_____

_____

_____

_____

D. She forgets to go to the bathroom and soils her underpants frequently. Sometimes, she becomes confused and doesn't know where the bathroom is located. Then she cries. What advice can you give?

_____

_____

_____

_____

E. The daughter says that she's heard about an Alzheimer's support group that meets each week in a nearby church hall. She asks you about the benefits of joining such a group. How will you reply?

_____

_____

_____

_____

_____

2. Mr. Yancy has been receiving a series of radiation treatments at the local medical center following cancer surgery. He returns home after each treatment. The next day he is exhausted and has no appetite. A transdermal patch on his upper arm gives medication to help relieve the severe pain in his back. During each visit you help him to take a partial bath at the bathroom sink, and you prepare his lunch and perform various housekeeping duties.

A. How will you help him with the partial bath?

_____

_____

_____

B. There are markings on his lower back where the radiation treatments are given. How will you care for this area?

_____

_____

_____

_____

C. What will you do to encourage him to eat?

_____

_____

_____

_____

D. List four conditions that you will report to your supervisor.

_____

_____

_____

_____

_____

3. Your client, Fernando, has acquired immunodeficiency syndrome. He lives alone in a two-room apartment and looks forward to your visit each day. Fernando spends a lot of time in bed because he has very little energy. In addition, he has the following symptoms:
    · Cough; brings up blood-tinged sputum
    · No appetite
    · Diarrhea about twice a week
    · 20-lb weight loss in the past 6 weeks
    · Bleeding gums
    · Swelling of the legs and ankles
    The care plan includes giving a complete bed bath, encouraging fluids, and keeping his feet elevated when out of bed.

A. Describe five special precautions you will take to control infection when caring for Fernando. Explain your reasons.

_____

_____

_____

_____

B. You notice that there are reddened areas on his elbows, heels, and lower back. What will you do?

_____

_____

_____

_____

C. When preparing meals for Fernando, list three precautions you will take to prevent infection.

_____

_____

_____

_____

_____

D. One day, while you are caring for Fernando, his sister comes to visit. She says to you, "You're very brave to be caring for my brother. Don't you worry that you'll get AIDS from him?" How will you answer this question?

_____

_____

_____

_____

E. She also tells you that she and her brother were always very fond of each other. "We were always hugging. Now, it's different. He's so sick—I'm afraid to even touch him." What is your response?

_____

_____

_____

_____

_____

4. Sara Turner had her gallbladder removed. She has returned home after one night in the hospital. She has a tube in her abdomen that is draining green liquid into a collecting bag, which is almost full. She needs to cough but is afraid to do so. She complains about pain in the area of the drain. You are her home care aide. What would you do about:

A. Drainage bag almost full?

_____

_____

B. Fear of coughing?

_____

_____

C. Pain in area of drainage tube?

_____

_____

5. Following a cerebrovascular accident, Mrs. Potts was transferred to the rehabilitation center where she learned to walk using a walker. She still has some difficulty chewing and swallowing and remembering the correct names of things. She is easily frustrated and cries when she tries to do something. How can you assist Mrs. Potts with:

A. Safe ambulation?

_____

_____

_____

_____

_____

B. Adequate nutrition?

_____
_____
_____
_____

C. Communication?

_____
_____
_____
_____

D. Emotional support?

_____
_____
_____
_____

6. Mr. Fugil was admitted to the medical center in an unconscious state. Tests revealed a very high blood glucose level. Diabetes mellitus was diagnosed. When he was discharged, a home care aide was assigned to assist him because he was very weak and needed help with personal care for a short time. The home care aide discovered that Mr. Fugil is not following the prescribed diet. He snacks on cake, cookies, cheese, and crackers. He has ice cream for dessert every night. He refuses to test his blood glucose and refuses to take his insulin. He says he doesn't like to "stick" himself. What should the home care aide do?

_____
_____
_____
_____

True or False

Directions: In the space provided, mark the statement "T" for true or "F" for false. If false, change the statement to make it true.

1. _____ Another name for stroke is cerebrovascular accident.
2. _____ Clients with chronic obstructive pulmonary disease have difficulty breathing.
3. _____ Edema is swelling of the tissues and is common in cardiovascular disease.
4. _____ Cancer is the second leading cause of death in the United States.
5. _____ Cancer treatment causes no side effects or problems.
6. _____ Parkinson's disease is an acute illness affecting young adults.
7. _____ Clients with multiple sclerosis often experience bladder problems.
8. _____ Postoperative clients are at risk for infection.
9. _____ Reasoning with an Alzheimer's client will help him/her to understand what is happening.
10. _____ An identification bracelet is important for the Alzheimer's client who wanders.
11. _____ Clients with circulatory problems tire easily.

12. _____ Human immunodeficiency virus causes AIDS.

13. _____ Diarrhea, malnutrition, and wasting are serious problems for clients with AIDS.

14. _____ Standard (universal) precautions are used only when caring for clients with AIDS.

15. _____ AIDS clients should not handle soiled cat litter or other animal bedding.

16. _____ The term *arthritis* means inflammation of the joints.

17. _____ The client with a cast can take a tub bath.

18. _____ It is normal for the client with a casted arm to have cold, blue fingers, that he or she cannot move.

19. _____ Always wear gloves when handling body fluids.

20. _____ Encourage clients to do as much as possible for themselves according to their condition.

21. _____ The home care aide may change sterile surgical dressings.

22. _____ "Phantom limb pain" following an amputation is all in the client's imagination.

23. _____ Clients with low energy levels should not be rushed through activities of daily living.

24. _____ Clients with poor appetites should be given big meals with lots of food.

25. _____ Many clients with chronic illness have a low self-image and are often frustrated and discouraged.

23

Caring for the Dying Client

Completion

Directions: Fill in the blank(s) with the appropriate word(s).

1. Emotional responses to dying are _____, _____, _____, _____, and _____.
2. A final illness from which a client is not expected to recover is called a _____ illness or an _____ disease.
3. Living will and durable power of attorney are examples of _____.
4. A program that cares for the dying client and his or her caregivers is _____.
5. Two signs of approaching death are _____ and _____.
6. The last sense to leave the body is _____.
7. Care given after death is called _____ care.

Situations

Directions: Read the situation and answer the questions on the lines provided.

1. Mr. Toomey has terminal cancer. He is no longer being treated for the disease and is being cared for in a hospice program. He asks you, "Am I going to die?" How would you respond?

_____

_____

_____

_____

2. Your client is very sad and quiet. She sleeps most of the day and does not want any company. Her family is very upset, and they feel she has given up and does not want to get well. What would you do?

_____
_____
_____
_____

3. Your client and caregivers keep hoping for a miracle cure for AIDS. They read medical journals and search computer websites in hope of learning about a cure. What is your feeling about their hope?

_____
_____
_____
_____

4. Josephine tells you that you are stupid and do everything wrong. She says, "You don't even know how to comb my hair right." You have been caring for this hospice client for 4 months. How would you answer her?

_____
_____
_____
_____

5. Even though you knew that your client was going to die, when it happened you were shocked. The next day, you feel very sad and cry about his death. How can you cope with these feelings?

_____
_____
_____
_____

6. Your client's wife tells you that after her husband dies, the elders of her religious community will bathe and dress the body in preparation for immediate burial. What should you do?

_____
_____
_____
_____

7. The Weinberg family wants to say "goodbye" to their dying mother, but they say it's too late because she is already unconscious. What would you tell them?

_____
_____
_____
_____

24

Emergencies

Completion

Directions: Complete the following sentences in the space provided.

1. The emergency telephone number to call in my area is _____.
2. The Poison Control Center's telephone number in my area is _____.
3. The four Cs of Emergency Care are _____, _____, _____, and
   _____.
4. First aid situations that increase the home care aide's risk for infection are _____,
   _____, and _____.
5. The four signs of a medical emergency that require immediate action are _____,
   _____, _____, and _____.

Situations (A)

Directions: For each of the emergency situations listed below, give four actions you will take besides calling for help.

1. Victim has severe bleeding from a wound on the right arm.
   A. _____
   B. _____
   C. _____
   D. _____
2. Victim appears gray and has cold, clammy skin; a weak, rapid pulse; and shallow respirations.
   A. _____
   B. _____
   C. _____
   D. _____

3. Client scalds left hand while pouring boiling water from a pan on the stove. The area is very red, and there are blisters forming on the skin.
   A. _____
   B. _____
   C. _____
   D. _____
4. Client tells you that she feels like she is going to have a seizure.
   A. _____
   B. _____
   C. _____
   D. _____
5. Victim is not breathing, cannot speak, has his hands around his neck, and is sitting in a chair.
   A. _____
   B. _____
   C. _____
   D. _____
6. Your client has fallen down the last three steps of the stairway. She is on her left side and complains of severe pain in her left leg and hip. Also, she cannot move her left wrist.
   A. _____
   B. _____
   C. _____
   D. _____
7. You are shopping at the local mall with your friend. Suddenly, he clutches his chest and says, "The pain is back. Now, it's in my left arm, too."
   A. _____
   B. _____
   C. _____
   D. _____

Situations (B)

Directions: Read the following situations and answer the questions.

1. While walking from the bus stop to your client's apartment, a woman runs toward you. Her coat is on fire. What will you do first?

   _____
   _____
   _____
   _____
   _____

2. Your aunt asks you to advise her about what items to buy for the family's first aid kit. List six items you will recommend.

A. _____

B. _____

C. _____

D. _____

E. _____

F. _____

3. You find Louisa, aged 3 years, in the bathroom, drinking toilet bowl cleaner. List two actions you will take.

A. _____

B. _____

Who will you call and what will you report?

_____

_____

_____

_____

4. Your client has been taken to the hospital by the emergency medical services personnel following a medical emergency. What information (list four) will you include when reporting and recording the emergency to your agency?

A. _____

B. _____

C. _____

D. _____

25

Part 5
Professional Skills

Getting a Job
and Keeping It

Crossword Puzzle

Directions: Complete the crossword puzzle by identifying important terms found in Chapter 25.

ACROSS

1. A person in a school who helps students find employment
4. Health insurance, life insurance, and a prescription plan
6. To receive a copy of the personnel policies and to keep records of your attendance
8. Recognition by a government agency that an individual has met certain requirements
10. A formal meeting between an employer and a job applicant
11. Matches job seekers and potential employers
12. Programs to help you to keep your skills up to date

DOWN

1. A form to be filled out when applying for a job
2. To perform your duties properly and to use the correct forms to record client care and billable time
3. Process of judging employee performance to determine suitability to remain on the job
5. Wages earned
7. Required
9. Informal method of exchanging information about job openings

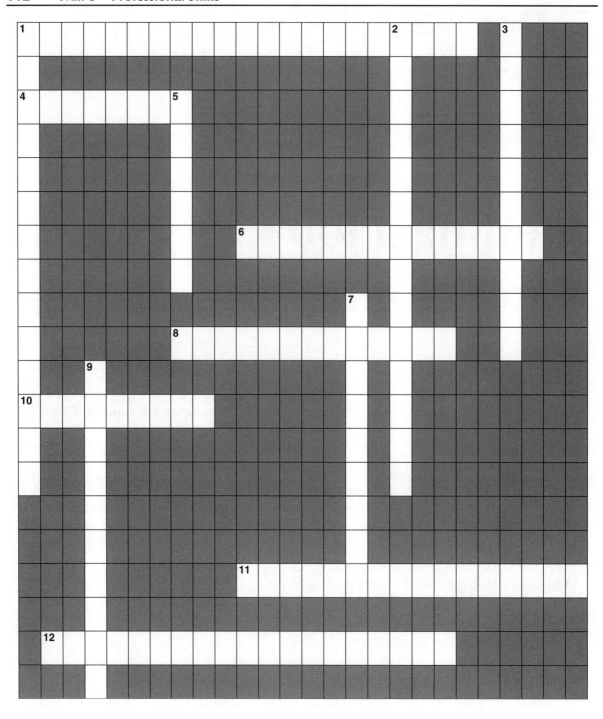

Want Ad

Directions: Read the want ad below and answer the questions

CERTIFIED HOME CARE AIDES
ABC Home Care Agency, Inc. is currently expanding services.
Exp. pref'd. Cert. req. Car req.
*M-F + wknd
*Live-in work
*Excel pay + benefits
*Travel reim.
Call for interview 000-123-4567

---

1. What do the following abbreviations mean?
   A. Exp _____
   B. Pref'd _____
   C. Cert. _____
   D. Req. _____
   E. Excel _____
   F. Reim. _____
2. What do the following terms mean?
   A. Travel reim.: _____
   _____
   _____
   B. M-F + wknd: _____
   _____
   _____
   C. Live-in work: _____
   _____
   _____
   D. Benefits: _____
   _____
   _____

3. Before calling the ABC Home Care Agency about the want ad, you prepare by
   A. _____
   B. _____

The Job Interview

Directions: Answer the questions in the space provided.

1. Your appointment to be interviewed by the personnel manager of ABC Home Care Agency is tomorrow at 1:30 PM. You should arrive at the agency no later than _____.
2. Complete the sample application form (Figure 25-1).
3. During the interview the personnel manager, Ms. Hanson, explained the responsibilities of certified home care aides as employees of the ABC Home Care Agency. She discussed work hours, pay, and benefits. She has not discussed travel requirements or uniforms. What will you do?

    _____

    _____

    _____

4. Ms. Hanson explains to you the rights of the ABC Home Care Agency. Under each "right" listed below, give two examples of how you will act.

    A. Right to expect that you will perform your duties properly
        1. _____
        2. _____
    B. Right to expect you to keep accurate records
        1. _____
        2. _____
    C. Right to expect you to use correct safety practices to protect yourself and your client
        1. _____
        2. _____
    D. Right to supervise and evaluate your performance
        1. _____
        2. _____

5. She also gives you information about your rights as an employee. Under each "right" listed below, give two examples of how your employer should act.

    A. Right to a safe working environment
        1. _____
        2. _____
    B. Right to be paid for the work you perform
        1. _____
        2. _____
    C. Right to be supervised properly
        1. _____
        2. _____
    D. Right to be evaluated regularly
        1. _____
        2. _____

APPLICATION FOR EMPLOYMENT
(Please print clearly)

Personal Information   Date: _____

Name _____
              Last   First   Middle

Address _____
         Street   City   State   Zip Code

Telephone _____ Social Security No. _____
     Area Code   Number

If under 18 years of age, do you have work permit?   ❑ Yes ❑ No

If not a U.S. citizen, do you have the right to remain permanently and work in the U.S.A.?   ❑ Yes ❑ No

    Alien Reg. No. _____

Employment Desired

Position applied for: _____

Shift you can work: ❑ Day ❑ Evening ❑ Either   Hours desired: ❑ Full time ❑ Part time ❑ Temporary

How did you learn of this opening? _____

Date you can start: _____
         Month   Day   Year

Have you ever applied to this company before? ❑ Yes ❑ No When _____

Have you ever worked for this company before? ❑ Yes ❑ No

When _____ Supervisor _____

Reason for Leaving _____
_____

Education

Highest grade completed (circle):   1 2 3 4 5 6 7 8   9 10 11 12   1 2 3 4
                    Grade School   High School   College

Name and location of last school attended _____

Vocational or trade training _____

Extracurricular
activities while in school _____

Area of specialization
or major interest _____

Professional organization memberships, honors received, volunteer or community service or other qualifications you have which you feel are related to the position for which you are applying:
_____
_____
_____
_____

Form 3290R BRIGGS, Des Moines, IA 50306 (800) 247-2343 PRINTED IN U.S.A.   Rev. 4/92

Figure 25-1

References

List three persons who know you well. Do not include relatives or former employers.

Name	Address	Phone	Years Acquainted With You

Former Employers

List below your work experience, starting with your present or last place of employment.

Date Employed	Name and Address of Employer	Name of Supervisor	Position(s) Held
from _____ to _____			start _____ finish _____
from _____ to _____			start _____ finish _____
from _____ to _____			start _____ finish _____
from _____ to _____			start _____ finish _____
from _____ to _____			start _____ finish _____

May we contact your present employer at this time?   ❑ Yes   ❑ No

Employment Understanding (Please Read and Sign)

This institution does not discriminate in hiring or any other decision on the basis of race, color, sex, citizenship, national origin, ancestry, Vietnam era veteran status, or on the basis of age or physical or mental disability unrelated to the ability to perform the work required. No question on this application is intended to secure information to be used for such discrimination.

I voluntarily give this institution the right to make a thorough investigation of my past employment and activities, agree to cooperate in such investigation and release from all liability or responsibility all persons, companies or corporations supplying such information. I consent to take the physical examination, and such future physical examinations as may be required by this institution at such times and places as the institution shall designate. I understand that an offer of employment may be contingent on passing the physical examination which relates to the essential duties I would be required to perform.

I understand that my employment is at will, and that either party is free to terminate the employment relationship at any time without cause. I also understand that my employment may be terminated for any misstatement or omission of fact appearing on this application form.

If employed, I will be required to complete an Employment Verification Form (1-9), and within three days show satisfactory evidence of identity and eligibility for employment.

_____   _____
Applicant's Signature   Date

Figure 25-1—Cont'd

6. Next to each of the behaviors listed below, place a "Yes" or "No" to indicate what is correct.

_____ A. Smoking

_____ B. Asking questions if you do not understand what the interviewer is saying

_____ C. Taking off your shoes because they are new and too tight

_____ D. Bringing your children with you

_____ E. Using your pen and paper to write down information that you want to remember

_____ F. Chewing gum

_____ G. Arriving early

_____ H. Thanking the interviewer for his or her time

_____ I. Keeping your cellular phone handly in case you get a call during the interview

Answers

ANSWERS

CHAPTER 1

Learning About Home Care

Matching

1. G
2. C
3. D
4. H
5. B
6. E
7. A
8. F

Situations

SITUATION 1

RESPONSE:

Length of course—this answer will be different for each program. Check with your teacher to make sure you have the correct answer for your training program.

Clinical experience—learning in the home of a client under the supervision of the instructor or home care nurse.

Evaluation—judging performance to determine progress in learning.

SITUATION 2

RESPONSE:

I want to do every thing I can do to learn. These are tools to help me do that job.

SITUATION 3

RESPONSE:

Suggest that your classmates tell the teacher what they don't understand. You go to the teacher and tell him or her that you didn't understand the "big words" and ask for help.

Practicing to Take Tests

TRUE OR FALSE

1. False. Home care aide programs vary from state to state. The word *all* makes this statement false.
2. True
3. True
4. False. Evaluating the home care aide's progress goes on throughout the entire program.
5. False. The client and the family help the instructor to evaluate the student's performance.
6. True

MULTIPLE CHOICE

1. b
2. c
3. a

Situations

Each person will have different answers and different schedules. Be prepared to discuss in class.

CHAPTER 2

The Home Care Industry

Matching

1. F
2. J
3. B
4. I
5. C
6. G
7. D
8. K
9. H
10. E
11. L
12. A
13. M

Hidden Words

```
C  E  V  I  T  A  R  E  P  O  O  C  E  P
O  O  E  T  R  E  L  A  P  R  I  O  N  L
M  P  N  L  O  W  I  L  T  T  L  U  T  E
P  A  R  S  B  G  E  N  S  S  U  T  S  A
E  T  L  T  I  A  E  A  C  E  F  N  U  S
T  I  A  B  S  D  I  H  C  N  T  A  O  L
E  E  E  A  I  S  E  L  L  O  C  V  E  U
N  N  N  F  U  E  R  R  E  H  E  R  T  F
T  T  N  H  R  A  K  L  A  R  P  E  R  L
L  O  T  F  E  S  D  I  N  T  S  S  U  L
C  N  U  W  I  L  L  I  N  G  E  B  O  I
E  L  B  A  D  N  E  P  E  D  R  O  C  K
S  I  N  C  E  R  E  G  N  I  R  A  C  S
```

Word Completion

1. Teaches client helpful hints to improve swallowing   Speech Therapist
2. Coordinates activities of the team   Case Manager
3. Supervises the activities of the LPN/LVN and home care aide   Registered Nurse
4. Gives spiritual guidance to the client   Clergy
5. Instructs the client and family about preparing meals according to the diet ordered by the doctor   Dietitian
6. Checks breathing equipment being used by the client   Respiratory Therapist
7. Arranges community services to be given   Social Worker
8. Provides complex nursing care to clients with special needs   Nurse Specialist
9. Gives personal care to clients and performs light housekeeping duties   Home Care Aide
10. Assesses the client's ability to perform ADL   Occupational Therapist
11. Gives nursing care to clients   Licensed Practical Nurse
12. Teaches exercises to strengthen leg muscles   Physical Therapist

True or False

1. T
2. F Never take your client's prescription drug.

3. F The physical therapist is responsible for evaluating his or her client's progress in physical therapy.
4. F After visitors arrive, keep yourself busy elsewhere in the home.
5. T
6. T
7. F It is important (necessary) to maintain healthy eating habits.
8. T
9. F Refuse the beer, politely.
10. F You do not agree to work extra hours. Ask the family to contact the agency about the need for more hours of service.

CHAPTER 3

Developing Effective Communication Skills

True or False

1. F Hearing impaired persons will understand what you are saying if you DO NOT exaggerate your words.
2. F It is helpful to keep a pad and pencil nearby so that your HEARING impaired client can communicate in writing, if necessary.
3. T
4. T
5. T
6. F Always stand IN FRONT of visually impaired clients because their side vision is NOT good.
7. T
8. F Speak in a NORMAL tone of voice to make sure your blind client understands what you are saying.
9. F While your client, Mr. Jackson, is asking you a question, be sure to concentrate on WHAT HE IS SAYING, NOT ON how you will answer him.
10. T
11. T
12. F The client does NOT have the right to refuse care given by an African American home care aide.
13. F You should NOT compliment her on how attractive she looks to make her feel better.
14. T
15. T

Situations

SITUATION 1
RESPONSE:

Mr. Walker, you wanted to talk about your wife's illness. Let's go into the living room. What did you want to tell me?

ACTION:

Do not go into the bedroom. Report this incident to your supervisor and prepare a written report.

SITUATION 2
RESPONSE:

I don't understand, Mr. D'Orio. What do you mean your son doesn't love you anymore?

ACTION:

Document what you have observed and what Mr. D'Orio has said. Report these observations to your supervisor.

SITUATION 3
RESPONSE:

I think you need more help than I can give to you. So, I'm notifying my supervisor immediately.

ACTION:

Go and call the supervisor.

SITUATION 4
RESPONSE:

It's very nice of you to think of me. But, I am not allowed to accept anything from my clients or their families.

ACTION:

Do not accept the money.

Matching

1. G
2. I
3. A
4. D
5. B
6. K
7. F
8. J
9. C
10. H
11. E

Diagram (Workbook Figure 3-1)

1. message
2. meaning
3. sender
4. receiver
5. feedback

Completion

1. Effective communication begins with the basic principle <u>respect for the client and family as human beings</u>.
2. Five ways to improve listening skills are:
   A. Be quiet
   B. Stop all other activities
   C. Listen to entire message
   D. Don't interrupt speaker
   E. Let speaker finish
   Other possibilities:
   Don't think of an answer while another is speaking
   Keep confidences
   Practice listening skills
3. Two topics to avoid when communicating with your client are <u>religion</u> and <u>politics</u>.
   Other possible answer: personal affairs of home care aide
4. Confidential information is shared with your supervisor when <u>it is necessary for the care, health, or well-being of client</u>.
5. To be a good listener, you must devote <u>your full attention</u> to the speaker.

CHAPTER 4

Understanding Your Client's Needs

Diagram (Workbook Figure 4-1)

1. physical
2. security and safety
3. love
4. self-esteem
5. self-actualization

Completion

A. Oxygen and food are examples of <u>physiological</u> need.
B. Preventing falls helps to meet a client's need for <u>safety</u>.
C. Feeling close to other persons helps to meet the need for <u>love</u>.
D. Feeling good about one's self is meeting the need for <u>self-esteem</u>.
E. By learning and creating, people meet their need for <u>self-actualization</u>.

True or False

1. <u>T</u>
2. <u>F</u> Families can include grandparents, grandchildren, stepchildren, stepparents, and others.
3. <u>T</u>
4. <u>T</u>
5. <u>T</u>
6. <u>F</u> Family members do *not* always work together to meet their own needs.
7. <u>F</u> The home care aide cannot meet all the needs of client and family.
8. <u>T</u>
9. <u>F</u> Everyone has personal needs.
10. <u>T</u>

Growth and Development

1. Many factors influence growth and development.
2. Early life experiences guide the foundation for our growth and development in later years.
3. Growth occurs in a logical pattern.
4. One stage of growth and development must be completed before moving on to the next stage.
5. Physical growth is completed around age 21, but emotional, social, and intellectual growth continues throughout life.

GROWTH AND DEVELOPMENT CHART *(Answers may vary—these are sample suggested answers.)*

Development Stage	Age	Characteristics	Ways to Meet Client Needs
Infancy	Birth	1. Tremendous growth	1. Hold and cuddle
	to 1 year	2. Learns to control head	2. Provide safe environment
		3. Learns to sit	3. Create dependable, loving, secure world
		4. Says first word	
		5. Begins to walk	
Toddler	1–3 years	1. Endless activity	1. Eliminate hazards
		2. Gets into everything; accident prone	2. Praise safe behavior
		3. Temper tantrums	3. Support parental toilet training program
		4. Plays alone	
Preschool	3–5 years	1. Endless energy	1. Avoid use of "don't"
		2. Eager to learn	2. Provide safe environment
		3. Imaginary playmates	3. Follow rituals for nap time, bed time, meals
		4. Rituals important	
School age	6–12 years	1. Slow, steady growth	1. Follow rules established in home
		2. Active, strong	2. Ensure adequate nutrition
		3. Enjoys friends	3. Respect privacy
		4. Likes challenges	4. Be honest
Adolescent	12–18 years	1. Rapid physical growth	1. Respect privacy
		2. Sexual maturation	2. Follow rules of home
		3. Striving for independence	3. Expect acceptable behavior
		4. Peers important	

Development Stage	Age	Characteristics	Ways to Meet Client Needs
Adulthood	18–65 years	1. Physical development completed	1. Maintain activities of daily living
		2. Career and financial independence	2. Offer choices in routine
		3. Parenting, bonding with partner	3. Involve in family life
Older adulthood	65–100+ years	1. Adjusting to physical changes	1. Provide safety
		2. Adjusting to retirement	2. Encourage independence
		3. Adjusting to death of partner	3. Allow time. Be calm and patient

CHAPTER 5

Understanding How the Body Works

Identification

ORGAN	SYSTEM
1. pituitary gland	endocrine
2. liver	digestive
3. prostate gland	male reproductive
4. bronchioles	respiratory
5. diaphragm	muscular
6. ribs	skeletal
7. arteries	circulatory
8. gallbladder	digestive
9. capillaries	circulatory
10. ovaries	female reproductive or endocrine
11. urethra	urinary
12. spinal cord	nervous
13. larynx	respiratory
14. brain	nervous

Fill in the Blanks

BODY SYSTEM	FUNCTION
1. skeletal	Provides support, protection, and movement
2. muscular	Allows movement
3. circulatory and lymphatic	Transports blood and tissue fluid throughout the body; fights infection
4. integumentary	Protects the body from injury
5. nervous	Sends and receives electrical messages and coordinates all body functions
6. respiratory	Takes in air and removes carbon dioxide from the body
7. endocrine	Produces hormones that regulate body functions
8. digestive	Responsible for nutrition and elimination of body waste
9. urinary	Filters all the blood to remove dissolved waste and excess water
10. reproductive	Responsible for production of offspring

Matching

1. I
2. D
3. E
4. H
5. G
6. J
7. C
8. B
9. F
10. A

Completion

1. Tissues are made up of groups of cells.
2. Another word for throat is pharynx.
3. Arteries carry blood from or away from the heart.
4. Capillaries connect arteries to veins.
5. A heart beat has two parts: contraction (systole) and relaxation (diastole).
6. A body system is made up of many organs.
7. Another word for windpipe is trachea.
8. The lid that prevents food from entering the respiratory system is the epiglottis.
9. The long, strong muscles are in the legs.
10. The urethra has two functions in the man because it carries urine and sperm.

Diagram

CIRCULATORY SYSTEM (WORKBOOK FIGURE 5-1)

1. heart
2. veins
3. arteries

RESPIRATORY SYSTEM (WORKBOOK FIGURE 5-2)

1. nose
2. pharynx
3. larynx
4. trachea
5. bronchus
6. lungs
7. alveoli

DIGESTIVE SYSTEM (WORKBOOK FIGURE 5-3)

1. mouth
2. pharynx
3. esophagus
4. stomach
5. small intestine
6. large intestine
7. liver
8. gallbladder
9. appendix
10. anal canal

CHAPTER 6

Observing, Reporting, and Recording

Matching

1. J
2. E
3. L
4. B
5. A
6. I
7. K

8. D
9. F
10. C
11. G
12. H

Reporting and Recording

1.	Bruise on client's arm	Record on client's record
2.	Client complains of sudden pain in chest	Notify supervisor immediately; record your observations and action taken
3.	Foul odor in refrigerator	Record your observations and action taken
4.	Severe difficulty in breathing	Notify supervisor immediately; record your observations and action taken
5.	Sudden vomiting and diarrhea	Notify supervisor immediately; record your observations and action taken
6.	Toilet overflowed—client lives alone; has no immediate family nearby	Notify supervisor immediately for directions
7.	Client refused lunch and drank one cup of tea	Record your observations and notify supervisor
8.	Client cried for half hour after brother's visit	Record your observations
9.	Client's daughter slapped her twice in the face during 15-minute visit	Record your observations and notify supervisor
10.	Client had been irritable but now is pleasant and talkative	Record your observations

True or False

1. T
2. F Care records are confidential and may not be shared with family members.
3. F Only a small portion of the record is in the home. Most of it is at the agency office.
4. T
5. T
6. T
7. F It is not the role of the Home Care Aide to change care plans.
8. T
9. T
10. F Call your supervisor whenever you feel it is necessary. It is always better to be safe rather than to say "I'm sorry" or "I thought."

Abbreviations

1. abd — abdomen/abdominal
2. ADL — activities of daily living
3. BP — blood pressure
4. Ca — cancer
5. meds — medication(s)
6. O_2 — oxygen
7. OOB — out of bed
8. ROM — range of motion
9. Tbsp — tablespoon
10. TPR — temperature, pulse, and respirations
11. $\bar{c}$ — with
12. ml — milliter
13. $\bar{s}$ — without
14. tsp — teaspoon

Recording (Workbook Figure 6-1)

See "Change in Condition" section, on pp. 132-133.

WEEKLY CLIENT CARE RECORD—CHANGE IN CONDITION

Date	Time	Observation	Action Taken
12/10/03	9:15 am	Client vomited breakfast.	Called supervisor. Called 9-1-1 and client's
		Feels dizzy. Skin blue.	sister. Ambulance took client and sister to
		Breathing is noisy.	hospital at 9:45 am. Mrs. Jones, supervisor came to home.

Signed: Your name, HCA

Checklist (Workbook Figure 6-1)

WEEKLY CLIENT CARE RECORD

Client _Sam Smith_
Address _123 Harmony Lane_
City _Anytown_ State _WV_ Zip _78412_
Phone (day) _____ (eve.) _____

Employee _Your name_
Title _Home Care Aide_
Soc. Sec. No. _912-01-5678_
Week Ending _6_ / _8_ _07_

Fill in the date for each day.

Write your initials in the box which corresponds to each task performed.

	DATE	6/2	6/3	6/4	6/5	6/6	6/7	6/8
	DAY	Mon.	Tue.	Wed.	Th.	Fri.	Sat.	Sun.
	TIME ARRIVED	9 am						
PERSONAL CARE:								
Bath ☐ Bed ☐ Chair ☑Shower ☐ Tub		YN						
Perineal Care								
Hair ☐ Groom ☐ Shampoo								
Mouthcare ☐ Denture Care								
Shave								
Nail Care ☐ Clean ☐ File								
Foot Care								
Special Skin Care								
Dressing ☑ Assist ☐ Complete		YN						
Toileting ☐ Bed Pan ☐ Commode								
Other instructions: _____								
CLIENT ACTIVITIES: Transfer Activity Instructions: _OOB to Chair_		YN						
Assist with walking ☐ Cane ☐ Walker ☐ Crutches								
Assist with exercises ☐ ROM ☐ Other (specify)								
Wheelchair activities								
Other instructions: _____								

(Continues)

	Mon.	Tue.	Wed.	Th.	Fri.	Sat.	Sun.
OTHER FUNCTIONS:							
Temp. ☐ Oral ☐ Rectal ☐ Underarm							
Pulse							
Respirations							
Blood Pressure							
Weigh Client	*yn*						
Record Intake/Output (use special form)							
OTHER FUNCTIONS:							
Prepare and serve meal/snack							
Special diet (Specify)							
Assist with feeding							
Medications reminder							
Ostomy care							
Incontinent care							
Record bowel movements							
Change in condition (office was notified)							
Other instructions:							
HOUSEHOLD SERVICES:							
Change/make client's bed	*yn*						
Clean client's room							
Clean bathroom	*yn*						
Clean kitchen; wash dishes							
Vacuum, sweep, dust							
Client laundry	*yn*						
Marketing							
Errands (specify)							
Other instructions:	*7*						
DEPARTURE TIME	*11am*						
TOTAL HOURS	*2hr.*						

I certify that the hours shown represent my true total hours worked.

Signature _____ *Your name* _____ Title _*Home Care Aide*_ Date _6/2/07_

Return form to Home Care Agency weekly.

Notify Home Care Agency if your client's condition has changed since your last visit.

Situations

1. Observe—find out about the indigestion. What does it feel like?
2. Report—call your supervisor.
3. Record—the indigestion, your call to the supervisor, and your actions.

Incident Report (Workbook Figure 6-2)

ABC Home Care Agency
INCIDENT REPORT

PERSON INVOLVED	(Last name) Your name/HCA	(First name)	(Middle initial)	Adult ☒	Child ☐	Male ☐	Female ☐	Age Your age

Address Your name/HCA

Date of incident/accident 0/0/00 Time of incident/accident 10 A.M. ☒ P.M. ☐ Exact location of incident/accident Bedroom ☐ Hallway ☐ Bathroom ☐ Other ☒ Specify client's porch

CLIENT List diagnosis if contributed to incident/accident: DNA
Client's condition before incident/accident: Normal ☐ Confused ☐ Disoriented ☐ Sedated ☐ (Drug ___ Dose ___ Time ___) Other ☐ Specify ___
Were bed rails ordered? Yes ☐ No ☐ Were bed rails present? Yes ☐ No ☐ If Yes, Up ☐ Down ☐ Was height of bed adjustable? Yes ☐ No ☐ If Yes, Up ☐ Down ☐

EMPLOYEE ☒ Name Your name/HCA Job title HCA Length of time in this position 1 year

VISITOR ☐ OTHER ☐ Home address Your address Home phone Your phone number

Occupation HCA Reason for presence assigned to care for client

Equipment involved ☐ Property involved ☐ Describe DNA Was person authorized to be at location of incident/accident? Yes ☒ No ☐

Describe exactly what happened... My left foot went through weak board on client's porch. Fell and scraped left leg and hurt ankle. Ankle became swollen and sore

Indicate on diagram location of injury: Temp. ___ Pulse. ___ Resp. ___ B.P. ___

TYPE OF INJURY
1. Laceration ☐
2. Hematoma ☐
3. Abrasion ☒
4. Burn ☐
5. Swelling ☒
6. None apparent ☐
7. Other (specify below) ☐

LEVEL OF CONSCIOUSNESS

Name of supervisor notified Supervisor's name Time of notification 10:10 A.M./P.M. Time of responded 10:10 A.M./P.M.

Name and relationship of family member notified DNA Time of notification A.M./P.M. Time of responded A.M./P.M.

Was person involved seen by a physician? Yes ☒ No ☐ Where Medical center Date 0/0/00 Time 11:30 A.M.☒ P.M.☐

Was first aid administered? Yes ☐ No ☐ Where Date Time A.M.☐ P.M.☐

Was person involved taken to a hospital? Yes ☒ No ☐ hospital name Medical center By whom Supervisor Date 0/0/00 Time 11:45 A.M.☒ P.M.☐

Name, title, address & phone no. of witness(es) Additional comments and/or steps taken to prevent recurrence:

SIGNATURE/TITLE/DATE
Person preparing report Your name/HCA 0/0/00
Supervisor Supervisor Signature 0/0/00

Case Manager
Administrator

INCIDENT REPORT

CHAPTER 7

Working With the Ill and Disabled
Client Reactions

1. A. Anger or frustration.
   B. Pick up the fork and say, "This has been a trying day for you. How can I help?"

2. A. Withdrawal.
   B. Ignore the behavior. Continue to prepare for her bed bath and talk to her, even if she does not respond.

3. A. Anxiety or fear.
   B. Encourage her to do the exercises. Reassure her that you are there to support her so she will not fall. Demonstrate what you would do if she begins to lose her balance.

4. A. Overdependence.
   B. Tell Sam that he needs to use his arm muscles for good circulation and to get strong again. Washing his own face is an easy way to begin.

5. A. Denial.
   B. Notify your supervisor immediately.

Family Situations

1. Tucker family:
   Listen to Mrs. Tucker. Explain that Mr. Tucker is angry about his illness, not angry at her. Mrs. Tucker's feelings are normal; others feel this way, too. Notify your supervisor regarding the conversation. Tell the supervisor what you have already said. Seek further advice. A caregiver support group might be helpful for Mrs. Tucker.
2. Ann Marie Burroughs:
   Listen carefully to what her mother is telling you. Tell her that you cannot provide the kind of assistance that might help Anne Marie and that you will call your supervisor for assistance. Call your supervisor and report what is happening.
3. Santiago family:
   Listen to Jose. Tell him that you will speak with your supervisor regarding his concerns. The agency will be able to refer him to people who can help him during this difficult period.

Crossword Puzzle

The crossword grid (answer key) contains the following filled answers:

- 1 Across: WITHDRAWN
- 2 Down: ANGER
- 4 Across: DEPRESSION
- 4 Down: DER
- 5 Down: ILLNESS
- 6 Across: ROLE
- 7 Across: DENIAL
- 8 Across: DISABILITY
- 9 Down: ANXIETY
- 3 Down: HEALTH
- 10 Across: OVERDEPENDENCE

CHAPTER 8

Maintaining a Safe Environment

Home Hazards (Workbook Figure 8-1)

1. Open closet door	1. Close door
2. Spill on floor	2. Wipe up spill
3. Magazines/newspaper on floor	3. Pick up magazines/newspaper
4. Appliance cord dangling	4. Place out of way
5. Pot holder next to working gas burner or stove	5. Remove pot holder

6. Toys on floor
7. Aerosol can near open flame
8. Food and cleaning supplies together
9. Poisons in reach of children
10. Knife within reach of children

6. Pick up toys
7. Remove and store properly
8. Separate and store properly
9. Store properly
10. Store properly

(Other appropriate answers acceptable)

Diagram (Workbook Figure 8-2)

1. Ingredient: fuel
   E.g., rubbish, oily rags, clothing, linens, towels, pot holders, paints, paint thinners, alcohol, perfumes, etc.
2. Ingredient: oxygen
   E.g., air, medical oxygen
3. Ingredient: heat source
   E.g., matches, cigarette lighters, pilot lights, faulty plugs and electrical wires, hair dryers, irons, curling irons, burning candles, lit cigarettes, cigars, pipes

Matching

1. <u>A</u> Fuel (and/or C [heat source] when lit and burning)
2. <u>C</u> Heat source
3. <u>A</u> Fuel
4. <u>B</u> Oxygen
5. <u>C</u> Heat source
6. <u>B</u> Oxygen
7. <u>B</u> Oxygen
8. <u>A</u> Fuel
9. <u>B</u> Oxygen
10. <u>C</u> Heat source
11. <u>A</u> Fuel
12. <u>A</u> Fuel

Situations

SITUATION 1

A. Personal safety rules
   1. <u>Be aware of her surroundings</u>
   2. <u>Walk confidently like she knows where she is going</u>
   3. <u>Carry a whistle, personal alarm</u>, or cellular telephone
   4. Use well-lighted bus stop that is used often
   5. Plan the shortest, safest route possible

6. Do not walk near doorways
7. Have exact change/token for bus in pocket
8. Walk near others
9. Wallet or purse not visible
B. Safety rules when riding a bus
  1. <u>Sit near the bus driver</u>
  2. <u>If she feels unsafe about getting off at the stop, ride to the next stop</u>
  3. <u>Do not talk to strangers</u>
  4. Be observant
C. Safety rules before reaching door to client's or her home
  1. <u>Have house key in her hand</u>
  2. <u>Don't go inside if she suspects that something is wrong</u>
  3. <u>Be aware of what is going on around her</u>
  4. Do not enter the elevator if she suspects anything is wrong—wait for the next elevator

SITUATION 2

A. Safety rules to follow to and from client's home
  1. <u>Keep your doors locked at all times</u>
  2. <u>Wear seat belt always</u>
  3. <u>Make sure you have at least a half tank of gas</u>
  4. <u>Never pick up hitchhikers</u>
  5. <u>Select most direct route</u>
  6. <u>Let your family know your route</u>
  7. <u>Let agency know when you leave home and arrive at client's home</u> (according to agency policy); carry your cellular telephone
  8. <u>Keep car in good repair</u>
  9. If car breaks down, do not get out
  10. Put on flashers
  11. If police arrive in unmarked car, ask for identification before opening window or door
  12. Place "Call Police" placard or sign in window and wait for police to arrive
  13. Do not leave car; stay in locked car and wait for police
  14. Keep purse or wallet out of sight

SITUATION 3

<u>Yes</u>	Blanket
<u>Yes</u>	Eating utensils
<u>No</u>	Pots and pans
<u>Yes</u>	Money, including coins
<u>Yes</u>	First aid kit
<u>Yes</u>	Extra car keys
<u>Yes</u>	Flashlight, including batteries
<u>Yes</u>	Important papers (e.g., insurance policies, wills)
<u>Yes</u>	Essential medications in childproof containers
<u>Yes</u>	Sweater
<u>Yes</u>	Canned food and can opener

<u>No</u>	Bottle of liquor
<u>Yes</u>	Bottle of water
<u>No</u>	Shampoo
<u>No</u>	Hair spray

CHAPTER 9

Maintaining a Healthy Environment

Household Tasks Schedule

Making client's bed	daily
Cleaning refrigerator	weekly
Cleaning commode	daily
Changing bed linens	weekly or as needed
Removing trash	daily
Laundering bed linens	weekly or as needed
Picking up clutter	daily
Washing dishes	daily
Dusting living room	weekly
Cleaning toilet and bathroom sink	daily
Sweeping kitchen floor	daily
Cleaning kitchen counters	daily

Cleaning and Storing Supplies

Dust cloths	Wash in soapy water and air dry
Broom	Shake into large moistened bag and hang
Sponges	Wash in soapy water and air dry
Bucket	Rinse and dry
Toilet brush	Rinse in cold water and store in container
Rubber utility gloves	Rinse exterior and air dry

Sorting Laundry

<u>D</u>	1. Dirty work clothes
<u>A</u>	2. White cotton athletic socks
<u>C</u>	3. Blue toilet lid cover
<u>A or C</u>	4. Cotton print sheets
<u>E</u>	5. Nylon underwear
<u>A</u>	6. White cotton sheets

B	7. Blue jeans
C	8. Light purple towels
B	9. Dark brown cotton tee shirt
C	10. Yellow jogging top and pants
A	11. Diapers
E	12. Pink embroidered sweater

True or False

1. F Sick people may be able to care for their own homes.
2. T
3. T
4. T
5. F Never use a sharp knife to remove frost from the refrigerator freezer.
6. F Do not wash wooden bowls in the automatic dishwasher.
7. T
8. T
9. T
10. T
11. T
12. T

CHAPTER 10

Meeting the Client's Nutritional Needs

Fill in the Blank

1. Food energy is measured by means of a unit called a <u>calorie</u>.
2. Carbohydrates are composed of the chemicals <u>carbon</u>, <u>hydrogen</u>, and <u>oxygen</u>.
3. Sugars and starches are examples of <u>carbohydrates</u>.
4. Amino acids are components of <u>proteins</u>.
5. Vitamins A, D, E, and K are <u>fat-soluble</u> vitamins.
6. A tool to use in menu planning is the <u>Food Guide Pyramid</u>.
7. Adults should eat <u>6 to 11</u> servings of food from the bread, cereal, rice, and pasta group.
8. Too much saturated fat may increase the level of <u>cholesterol</u> in the blood.
9. Roughage is another word for <u>fiber</u>.
10. The term used to describe poor appetite is <u>anorexia</u>.
11. When assisting a blind client to eat, the plate is described as a <u>clock</u>.
12. Foods high in salt are eliminated on the <u>sodium</u>-restricted diet.
13. Spicy, highly seasoned, and fried foods are omitted in the <u>bland</u> diet.

14. The human body is <u>60</u> percent fluid.
15. The daily need for water (fluids) is at least <u>1 quart or 4 to 6 cups or 1000 to 1500 ml</u>.
16. Lack of fluid in the body can cause <u>dehydration</u>.
17. Three factors to consider in menu planning are <u>food preferences</u>, <u>meal patterns</u>, <u>variety and/or moderation in intake; balanced diet</u>, and <u>adequate fluids</u>.
18. Butter, cream, and ice cream would be omitted on a <u>low-fat or low-cholesterol</u> diet.
19. Proper storage is essential to preserve the <u>quality</u> and <u>safety</u> of foods.
20. Calcium and phosphorus are examples of <u>minerals</u> found in food and needed by the human body.

Crossword Puzzle

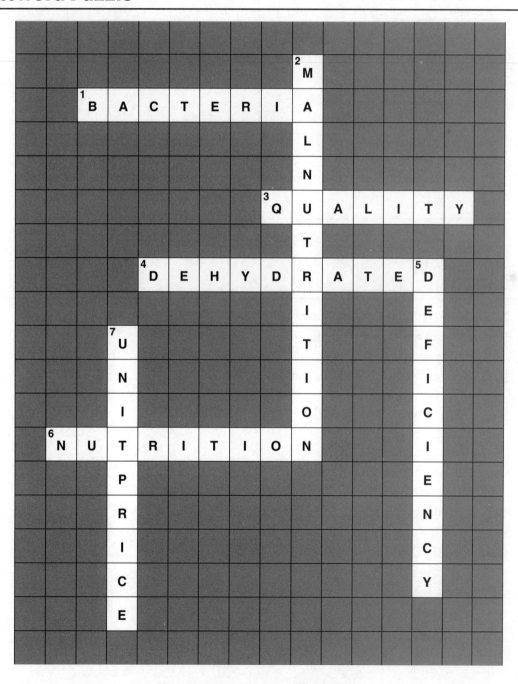

Food Guide Pyramid (Workbook Figure 10-1)

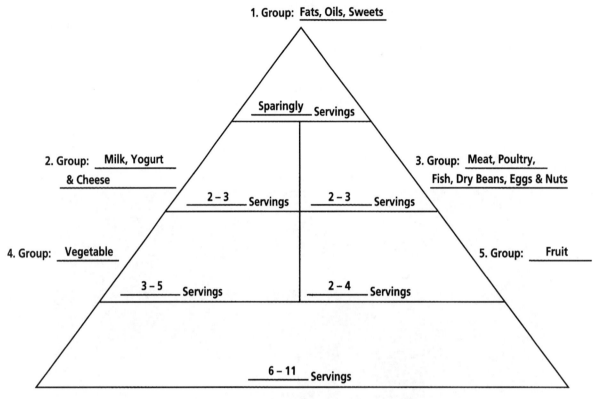

1. Group: **Fats, Oils, Sweets**

Sparingly Servings

2. Group: **Milk, Yogurt & Cheese**

2 – 3 Servings

3. Group: **Meat, Poultry, Fish, Dry Beans, Eggs & Nuts**

2 – 3 Servings

4. Group: **Vegetable**

3 – 5 Servings

5. Group: **Fruit**

2 – 4 Servings

6 – 11 Servings

6. Group: **Bread, Cereal, Rice & Pasta**

Matching

1. <u>A</u>, <u>B</u>, <u>C</u> Avoid serving crackers
2. <u>D</u> Prepare attractive, colorful meals
3. <u>A</u> Use drinking straws
4. <u>A</u>, <u>B</u>, <u>C</u> Avoid celery stalks and raw carrots
5. <u>C</u> Serve thick, soft foods
6. <u>A</u>, <u>B</u>, <u>C</u> Cut food into small pieces
7. <u>C</u> Use thickeners in fluids
8. <u>A</u> Use lightweight cups, glassware
9. <u>D</u> Serve fluids about 1 hour before meals
10. <u>A</u> Cut meat, butter bread
11. <u>D</u> Prepare small meals and snacks
12. <u>C</u> Add gelatin to cold liquids
13. <u>A</u>, <u>B</u>, <u>C</u>, <u>D</u> Allow plenty of time to eat

Therapeutic Diets (Workbook Figure 10-2)

The diets listed below are not meant to be the *only* correct answers, but are intended to give you an idea of the changes or substitutions you will need to make for clients who have diet restrictions.

A REGULAR	B HIGH FIBER	C LOW SODIUM	D LOW FAT/LOW CHOLESTEROL
Canned or Homemade Soup	Canned or Homemade Pea, Bean, or Vegetable Soup	Low-Sodium Canned or Homemade Soup	Low-Fat Canned or Homemade Soup
Ham Sandwich on Bread	Turkey Sandwich on Whole Wheat Bread	Low-Salt Turkey Sandwich on Bread	Low-Fat Turkey Breast on Reduced-Calorie Bread
Mayonnaise	Mayonnaise or Mustard		Mustard or Low-Fat Mayonnaise
Lettuce and Tomato	Lettuce and Tomato	Lettuce and Tomato	Lettuce and Tomato
Whole Milk	Whole Milk	Low-Fat/Fat-free Milk	Low-Fat/Fat-free Milk
Cookies	Fresh Fruit	Fresh Fruit	Fresh Fruit

Situations

SITUATION 1

Milk	amount; type (fat-free, 1%, 2%, evaporated)
Bread	amount; type (white, whole wheat, etc.)
Orange juice	amount; frozen, fresh, or concentrate; pulp, no pulp, added calcium
Eggs	amount; white or brown
Chopped beef	amount; type (chuck, round, fat content)
Carrots	amount; fresh, frozen, or canned
Bananas	amount; type; size; color
Broccoli	amount; fresh or frozen
Toilet paper	amount; color; brand name
Ice cream	amount; flavor; brand name; type (fat free, ice milk, frozen yogurt, etc.)

A N S W E R S

SITUATION 2

Milk	refrigerator
Bread	refrigerator or pantry
Orange juice	refrigerator or freezer
Eggs	inside refrigerator, not door
Chopped beef	refrigerator for immediate use, otherwise freeze
Carrots	refrigerator
Bananas	pantry
Broccoli	refrigerator or freezer
Toilet paper	bathroom closet or pantry
Ice cream	freezer

SITUATION 3

RESPONSE:

Tell Mrs. Smith you cannot take her anywhere without following the agency's rules.

ACTION:

Notify your supervisor.

CHAPTER 11

Preventing Infection/Medical Asepsis

Matching

1. F
2. G
3. C
4. K
5. A
6. D
7. I
8. L
9. B
10. H
11. E
12. J

True or False

1. T
2. F Standard (universal) precautions are used for all clients.

3. F When in doubt about disinfecting items in the home, ask your supervisor.
4. T
5. F　Microorganisms are found everywhere.
6. T
7. F OSHA regulations concerning bloodborne pathogens must be followed by anyone who may come in contact with blood and other body fluids.
8. T
9. T
10. T

Completion

1. To grow and multiply, all microorganisms need <u>moisture</u>, <u>warmth</u>, and <u>food</u>; or <u>host</u>, <u>darkness</u>, and <u>oxygen</u>.
2. Boil items for <u>20</u> minutes to destroy pathogenic organisms.
3. When preparing vinegar solution, use <u>one</u> part vinegar to <u>three</u> parts water.
4. Disinfection using the oven requires that items be baked for <u>1 hour</u> at a temperature of <u>350°F (180°C)</u>.
5. When preparing bleach solution, use <u>one</u> part bleach to <u>ten</u> parts water.
6. Bleach solution must be put in a plastic container. The label must contain this information: <u>name of solution (bleach)</u>, <u>strength (1:10)</u>, and <u>date</u>.
7. Handwashing is required <u>before</u> giving client care and <u>after</u> giving client care.
8. The most common household disinfecting solution is <u>soap</u> or <u>detergent</u> and <u>hot water</u>.
9. Microorganisms can be transmitted by means of <u>food</u>, <u>water</u>, <u>insects</u>, <u>direct or indirect human contact</u>, <u>animals</u>, <u>air</u>.
10. Factors that help to increase the risk for infectious diseases include:
    A. <u>Age</u>
    B. <u>Great stress</u>
    C. <u>Poor living conditions</u>
    D. <u>Chronic or acute illness</u>
    E. <u>Poor nutrition</u>

Situations

1. As you remove the linens from your client's bed, you are stuck by an uncapped needle on an insulin syringe that has been accidentally left in the bed. What would you do?
<u>Wash your hands</u>.
<u>Cleanse the wound with antiseptic</u>.
<u>Notify your supervisor immediately</u>.
2. Mr. Werts is coughing up sputum and spitting it into an old coffee can. He wants you to empty the can into the toilet and return it to him. What would you do?
<u>Remove the can and discard</u>.
<u>Wash your hands</u>.
<u>Give him a box of tissues, teach him to cough into the tissue, and discard the tissue into a plastic bag</u>.
<u>Discuss with your supervisor</u>.

3. Mrs. Hunt uses two disposable insulin syringes a day. She also uses four lancets (short pointed blades) to collect blood to test her sugar level. How would these "sharps" be safely discarded? Mrs. Hunt should discard these in the following manner:
<u>Discard in plastic milk jug</u>.
<u>Discard in coffee can</u>.
<u>Discard according to agency/community policy</u>.

4. Your client has had an "accident" in bed. The client, his clothing, and the linens are soiled with urine and feces. Describe:
Protective equipment you would use:
<u>Gloves, plastic apron</u>
How you would transport soiled clothing and linen to the laundry area in the basement of the home:
<u>Plastic bag</u>
How you pretreat and launder soiled linens:
<u>Using gloves, remove and wash away any solid material with cold water, rinse, and then wash in hot water with detergent and bleach</u>

Cycle of Infection (Workbook Figure 11-1)

1. Pathogenic Organism
2. Reservoir
3. Exit from reservoir
4. Method of transmission
5. Entrance into a new host
6. Host

CHAPTER 12

Body Mechanics

Procedures

1. **Applying a transfer gait belt**
   <u>4</u>   Apply belt over clothing and around waist.
   <u>5</u>   Place belt buckles off center in front or back.
   <u>1</u>   Explain what you are going to do.
   <u>2</u>   Wash your hands.
   <u>3</u>   Assist client to sit on side of bed.
   <u>6</u>   Tighten belt until it is snug.

2. **Transferring from bed to chair/wheelchair — standing transfer**
   <u>3</u>   Lock brakes and place footrests out of the way.
   <u>1</u>   Wash your hands.
   <u>4</u>   Assist client to sit at side of bed.

_6_ Have client reach back and grasp the farthest armrest of the wheelchair with one hand, then the nearest armrest.

_2_ Place wheelchair parallel to bed on client's strong side.

_5_ Place your arms under client's arms and around client's back, locking fingers together.

3. Assisting client to sit on side of bed

_2_ Provide privacy.

_6_ Assist client to put on robe and footwear.

_3_ Lock wheels on bed or push bed against wall if there are no brakes.

_4_ Place client in Fowler's position.

_5_ On count of "3", shift your weight to back leg and slowly swing client's legs over edge of bed while pulling shoulders to sitting position.

_1_ Explain what you are going to do.

4. Raising client's head and shoulders

_1_ Explain what you are going to do.

_4_ Slip your farthest arm under client's neck and shoulders.

_6_ Rock client to a semi-sitting position.

_2_ Wash your hands.

_3_ Lower head of bed and remove pillows.

_5_ Lock arms with client on side nearest you.

5. Moving client to side of bed

_1_ Explain what you are going to do.

_4_ Place arms underneath client.

_5_ Move client in three segments from center of bed to the edge.

_3_ Stand with feet apart.

_6_ Shift weight from front leg to back leg when moving client.

_2_ Wash your hands.

Identify the Incorrect Posture

1. (Figure 12-1) Bend at the knees to pick up box.
2. (Figure 12-2) Stand up straight with shoulders back. Pull in stomach muscles.
3. (Figure 12-3) Move walker closer to body so that all legs are on the floor. Encourage client to stand erect, wear study shoes, and belt robe.

Matching

1. E
2. I
3. D
4. J
5. B
6. A
7. H
8. C

9. G
10. F

Situations

1. <u>Explain that there is an easier and safer way to get out of bed</u>. <u>Demonstrate the procedure</u>.
2. <u>Make her comfortable on the floor and call your supervisor immediately</u>.

Identifying the Position

1. Figure 12-4 (Prone)
2. Figure 12-5 (Sims')
3. Figure 12-6 (Lateral or side-lying)
4. Figure 12-7 (Supine)
5. Figure 12-8 (Fowler's)

Safety Factors

1. Use wide base of support.
2. Wear flat/low-heeled shoes.
3. Use long muscles of arms and legs.
4. Keep back straight.
5. Have a plan of action.
6. Lock brakes on bed/wheelchair.
7. Adjust bed to convenient working height (or kneel or squat).
8. Have client help as much as possible so you don't have to do all the work.
9. Client wears shoes.
10. Use transfer belt to assist.

CHAPTER 13

Bedmaking

Diagram (Workbook Figure 13-1)

A. blanket
B. drawsheet
C. pillowcase
D. top sheet
E. bottom sheet

True or False

1. <u>T</u>
2. <u>T</u>
3. <u>T</u>
4. <u>T</u>
5. <u>F</u> Do not use a dry cleaner's bag because it can be harmful to the client.
6. <u>F</u> An occupied bed is made while the client remains in bed.
7. <u>T</u>
8. <u>T</u>
9. <u>F</u> Do not shake linens at any time.
10. <u>T</u>
11. <u>F</u> Hold linens away from your clothing.
12. <u>T</u>
13. <u>T</u>
14. <u>F</u> The most important reason for making a clean, neat, wrinkle-free bed is for the client's comfort.
15. <u>F</u> Do not wash the egg crate foam mattress. Washing will remove the fireproofing. Discard soiled foam mattress and replace.

CHAPTER 14

Personal Care

Procedures

1. Giving a back rub

<u>6</u> Remove excess lotion with towel.
<u>3</u> Place client on side or abdomen to expose entire back.
<u>2</u> Remove clothing from upper body.
<u>4</u> Rub hands together to warm lotion.
<u>5</u> Use long, firm, but gentle strokes—up, out, and down.
<u>1</u> Provide privacy (close door, shut drapes, pull shades).

2. Giving a complete bed bath

<u>5</u> Wash the genital and rectal areas.
<u>4</u> Give a back rub.
<u>6</u> Remove soiled towel and washcloth and place in area to be washed.
<u>3</u> Wash and dry leg while other foot is soaking.
<u>1</u> Obtain materials.
<u>2</u> Wash eye areas gently with clean water only.

3. Giving a shower in the bathtub

<u>4</u> Adjust water temperature and water pressure.
<u>5</u> Assist client into tub and to use grab bars.
<u>6</u> Clean tub and remove towels to area to be washed.

<u>2</u> Place nonskid mat in tub.
<u>3</u> Place bath chair in tub.
<u>1</u> Check temperature of bathroom for warmth and to see that it is free of drafts.

4. Shaving the male client using a blade razor

<u>1</u> Explain what are you going to do.
<u>3</u> Put on gloves.
<u>4</u> Wet and lather client's face.
<u>6</u> Remove gloves and wash your hands.
<u>5</u> Shave in direction of hair growth.
<u>2</u> Obtain materials.

5. Caring for client's hair

<u>4</u> Brush hair, section by section, from root to end of hair.
<u>1</u> Explain what you are going to do.
<u>2</u> Wash your hands.
<u>3</u> Place bath towel around client's shoulders.
<u>6</u> Wash your hands.
<u>5</u> Arrange hair as client wishes.

6. Caring for dentures

<u>3</u> Assist client to remove dentures from mouth.
<u>2</u> Wash your hands and put on gloves.
<u>4</u> Fill sink with warm water.
<u>6</u> Assist client to replace dentures in mouth.
<u>5</u> Brush dentures with toothpaste and rinse.
<u>1</u> Obtain materials.

True or False

1. <u>F</u> Personal care is given according to the care plan.
2. <u>T</u>
3. <u>F</u> Dentures are cleaned with warm water and toothpaste.
4. <u>T</u>
5. <u>T</u>
6. <u>T</u>
7. <u>F</u> The chair should have suction cups at the base of the legs.
8. <u>T</u>
9. <u>T</u>
10. <u>T</u>
11. <u>F</u> Weights are not used; deep knee bends are not done. Joints are taken through normal range of motion.
12. <u>T</u>
13. <u>F</u> Encourage clients to perform self-care as much as possible.
14. <u>T</u>
15. <u>T</u>

What Needs To Be Corrected

1. A. Aide is not wearing gloves; no towel across client's chest; hand should not be on client's head.
   B. Aide <u>must wear</u> gloves; place towel on client; move aide's hand from client's head.
2. A. Dentures, hearing aids, and eyeglasses are not properly stored. Urinal should not be on bedside stand.
   B. Put dentures in a cup with lid; put hearing aids in proper storage container; put eyeglasses in case and place in drawer. Urinal needs to be emptied and not placed near drinking glass. Store urinal properly.
3. A. Bedpan should not be on floor.
   B. Bedpan should be stored out of sight.
4. A. Bed linens should not be placed on the floor.
   B. Place linens in a laundry basket.
5. A. Side rails are down.
   B. When client is in bed with bed at highest level, side rails should be up.

CHAPTER 15

Elimination

Procedures

1. Giving and removing a bedpan

3   Give toilet paper and ask client to call when finished.
4   Place client in flat position and remove bedpan.
1   Raise bed to convenient working height.
5   Cleanse perineal area with toilet tissue, if necessary, wiping from front to back.
2   Warm bedpan with warm tap water. Dry with paper towels.
6   Cover bedpan, take to bathroom, and empty contents.

2. Giving and removing a urinal

2   Give urinal to client so he can position it properly.
6   Help client to wash hands.
4   Rinse urinal with cold water; clean and disinfect.
3   Put on gloves and remove urinal.
1   Assist client to stand.
5   Put urinal away; remove and discard gloves.

3. Care of the client with an indwelling catheter

6   Record what you have done and report any abnormal conditions.
1   Put on gloves.
4   Tape and position catheter properly.
2   Give perineal care.

<u>5</u>   Remove plastic drawsheet or incontinence pad.

<u>3</u>   Wash catheter tube in a downward motion away from the urinary meatus for approximately 4 inches (20 cm).

4. Applying a condom catheter

<u>1</u>   Put on gloves.

<u>5</u>   Connect catheter tip to drainage tubing.

<u>3</u>   Give perineal care.

<u>6</u>   Remove and discard gloves.

<u>2</u>   If condom catheter is present, remove gently and place in plastic bag.

<u>4</u>   Hold penis firmly and roll condom catheter onto penis with drainage opening at the urinary meatus.

What Needs To Be Corrected

1. A. Foley bag is above bladder (Extra credit—client has bare feet)
   B. Lower the bag (Extra credit—put shoes on client's feet)
2. A. Catheter tubing is dangling and collection bag is on side rail
   B. Properly pin tubing to the bottom sheet and position bag on bed frame
3. A. Client is wearing leg bag in bed
   B. Remove leg bag and connect to regular drainage bag and tubing
4. A. Collection bag is hanging on the wrong side of the side rail
   B. Move collection bag to hang freely behind side rail
5. A. Catheter tubing is kinked
   B. Straighten tubing and make sure it is properly pinned to bottom sheet. Position collection bag properly.

Situations

1. I = <u>600</u> ml
   O = <u>375</u> ml and one small <u>bowel movement</u> (BM)
2. <u>Know client's bowel habits and assist to commode immediately</u>.
   <u>Encourage the client to drink water and other fluids and to eat high-fiber foods</u>.
   <u>Do not have her wait when she has an urge to have a BM</u>.
   <u>Provide privacy</u>.
3. <u>Notify your supervisor of the situation</u>.
   <u>Clean skin with soap and warm water. Rinse and dry thoroughly</u>.
4. A. <u>Tell the companion that you will notify your supervisor</u>.
   B. <u>Give skin care to the client</u>.
   <u>Dispose of fecal matter from the pouch</u>.
   <u>Clean the pouch</u>.

Completion

1. Three characteristics of normal urine are <u>light yellow</u>, <u>clear</u>, and <u>slightly acid odor</u>.
2. Two characteristics of a normal BM are <u>light to dark brown</u> and <u>semi-solid</u>.

3. The medical term to describe air or gas in the intestine that is passed through the rectum is <u>flatus</u>.
4. Two kinds of gas-forming foods are <u>beans</u> and <u>cabbage</u>.
5. When clients are not able to control urination and/or bowel movements, the medical term to use is <u>incontinent or incontinence</u>.
6. If you notice changes in your client's urine or bowel movements, notify <u>your supervisor</u>.
7. Your client has not had a BM for more than 1 week and complains of abdominal discomfort. Also, you notice that small amounts of fecal liquid leak out of the anus. These may be signs that your client has a <u>fecal impaction</u>.
8. Waste materials are eliminated from the body by <u>perspiration from skin</u>, <u>urine</u>, <u>carbon dioxide and moisture from the lungs</u>, and <u>bowel movements</u>.
9. The medical term for material eliminated from the large intestine is <u>feces</u>.
10. The medical term to describe the process of eliminating solid waste through the anus is <u>defecation</u>.
11. When waste products in the large intestine move so rapidly that water is not able to be absorbed, the term used is <u>diarrhea</u>.
12. When providing perineal care or removing a bedpan, it is important to <u>wear disposable gloves</u>.
13. Three ways to help clients to maintain normal urination are:
    A. <u>Provide privacy</u>
    B. <u>Give them enough time to urinate</u>
    C. <u>Position them in normal voiding position</u>

CHAPTER 16

Collecting Specimens

Procedures

1. **Collecting a routine urine specimen**
   3 Pour urine into graduate and then into specimen container until 3/4 full.
   1 Label container.
   6 Store specimen in refrigerator.
   2 Have client void into commode, bedpan, urinal, or "hat."
   4 Put lid on specimen container.
   5 Remove and discard gloves.

2. **Collecting a stool specimen**
   1 Explain what you are going to do.
   4 Transfer stool to specimen container using tongue depressor.
   2 Label container.
   3 Put on gloves.
   6 Record what you have done and report any abnormal conditions to your supervisor.
   5 Flush remaining feces down toilet and assist client to complete toileting, as necessary.

3. Collecting a sputum specimen

<u>5</u>   Place container into plastic bag, then into paper bag.
<u>3</u>   Have client hold sputum specimen container.
<u>6</u>   Remove and discard gloves.
<u>1</u>   Obtain materials.
<u>4</u>   Do not touch the inside of the container. Keep the outside clean and free of any sputum.
<u>2</u>   Assist client to rinse mouth with plain water.

True or False

1. <u>T</u>
2. <u>F</u> Have client discard used lancets according to agency policy and community policy.
3. <u>F</u> Label specimen container as follows: client's name, address, date, and time of specimen collection.
4. <u>T</u>
5. <u>T</u>
6. <u>T</u>
7. <u>F</u> Fill container only ¾ full.
8. <u>F</u> Always wear gloves when collecting specimens.
9. <u>F</u> Collect 2 tablespoons of stool.
10. <u>F</u> When collecting this 24-hour urine specimen, discard the 3 P.M. Thursday specimen. Then save all urine during the 24-hour period including the voided specimen at 3 P.M. on Friday.

Crossword Puzzle

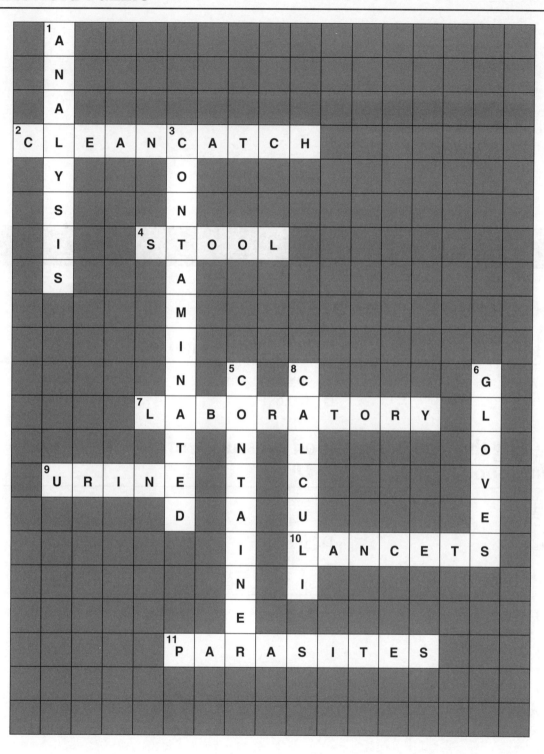

What Needs To Be Corrected

1. A. Label on lid, not container
   B. Place label on container
2. A. Container is too full
   B. Discard some of the specimen so container is 3/4 full
3. A. Ungloved hand
   B. Put gloves on
4. A. Incomplete information on label
   B. Complete information needed

CHAPTER 17

Measuring Vital Signs

Reading the Thermometer (Workbook Figures 17-1 *A-F*)

A. 97° F
B. 100.8° F

C. 99.2° F
D. 102.6° F

E. 98.4° F
F. 101.2° F

Reading the Dial of the Blood Pressure Cuff (Workbook Figures 17-2 *A-D*)

A. $\frac{110}{72}$

B. $\frac{126}{92}$

C. $\frac{220}{94}$

D. $\frac{168}{78}$

Matching

1. J
2. M
3. K
4. L
5. I
6. A
7. N
8. E
9. G
10. F
11. O
12. B
13. D

14. H
15. C

Reporting Vital Signs

1. _✗_ T. 103.2° F (O) (39.5° C)
2. ___ P. 72, regular
3. ___ T. 98.6° F (O) (37° C)
4. _✗_ R. 10 with wheezing and pain
5. _✗_ P. 123, weak
6. ___ T. 99.5° F (T) (37.5° C)
7. ___ BP 118/70
8. _✗_ BP 220/94
9. _✗_ BP 70/30
10. _✗_ R. 16, periods of no breathing, then rapid breathing
11. ___ T. 99.6° F (O) (37.5° C)
12. _✗_ P. 69, irregular
13. ___ T. 96.8° F (A) (36° C)
14. ___ T. 100.6° F (R) (38.1° C)
15. _✗_ T. 102.2° F (O) (39° C)

Completion

1. Vital signs give important information about the body processes of <u>circulation</u>, <u>breathing</u>, and <u>heat regulation</u>.
2. Take the client's vital signs when the client is <u>resting</u>.
3. Factors that cause vital signs to increase are <u>exercise</u>, <u>age</u>, and <u>illness</u> (other answers include pain, medications, and fear).
4. Heat leaves the body by means of <u>exhaling</u> and <u>urine</u>.
5. It is 9:30 AM. Your client has just had a big cup of hot coffee. Take the oral temperature at <u>9:45 AM</u>.
6. Have the client hold the glass thermometer in the mouth for <u>3</u> minutes before you remove and read the thermometer.
7. To read the glass thermometer, hold it at <u>eye</u> level.
8. Remove the electronic thermometer and read the digital display window when you hear the "<u>beep</u>."
9. Read the <u>last</u> dot to change color on the disposable thermometer.
10. Your client has diarrhea. Do not take a <u>rectal</u> temperature.
11. The "normal" systolic pressure in an adult is <u>120</u>. The "normal" diastolic pressure in an adult is <u>80</u>.
12. The normal range of TPRs in adults is:
    T (O) <u>97.6°-99.6° F (36.5°-37.5° C)</u>
    P <u>60–100</u>
    R <u>12-20</u>

13. Before and after using the stethoscope, clean earpieces and chestpiece to prevent <u>spread</u> of <u>pathogens</u>.

14. Shake down the oral glass thermometer to <u>95° F (35° C)</u> before placing it under the client's tongue.

15. When cleaning the rectal thermometer, begin at the <u>stem</u>, and wipe <u>downward</u> toward the <u>bulb</u>. Use a <u>twisting</u> motion.

16. Do not use your <u>thumb</u> to take your client's pulse.

17. You begin to take your client's pulse at 10:35 AM. You finish taking this pulse at <u>10:36 AM</u>. You continue holding the pulse while you take the respirations. You finish taking the respirations at <u>10:37 AM</u>.

CHAPTER 18

Special Procedures

Situation

SITUATION 1

A. <u>Put gauze or cotton balls between the straps and the ears.</u>
   <u>Apply water-soluble lubricant around the nostrils.</u>
   <u>Offer fluids frequently.</u>
   <u>Put water-soluble lubricant on her lips.</u>
   <u>Give frequent oral hygiene.</u>
B. <u>Remove matches, lighters, cigarettes, or cigars from the area.</u>
   <u>Place "No Smoking" sign in Olga's room where oxygen is being used.</u>
   <u>Have an exit plan in case of fire.</u>
   <u>Know location of fully charged, working fire extinguisher.</u>
   <u>Place "No Smoking" sign on entrance door to Olga's home.</u>

SITUATION 2

A. <u>Red skin.</u>
   <u>Blisters on the skin.</u>
   <u>Client complains of burning sensations in area.</u>
   <u>Client complains of pain in area.</u>
B. <u>Check the skin every 10 minutes. Diabetics are at risk for burns.</u>
C. <u>Record what you have observed on the client care record.</u>
   <u>Notify your supervisor for further directions.</u>

SITUATION 3

A. <u>Explain that, according to state law, you are not permitted to give any medications or injections. Vitamins are drugs.</u>
B. <u>Notify your supervisor.</u>

SITUATION 4

A. <u>Ask Mrs. Choi to tell you more about her leg cramps. Tell her that you must report her symptoms to your supervisor. This way, she may get relief and not have to be uncomfortable.</u>
B. <u>Notify your supervisor immediately.</u>
C. <u>Do not permit the client to take the medication.</u>
   <u>Notify your supervisor.</u>

Procedures

1. Giving a sitz bath

<u>2</u>   Ask client to void.
<u>3</u>   Place sitz bowl so that drainage holes are at the back of the toilet.
<u>1</u>   Ask client to remove and discard dressing or pad, if worn. Assist, if needed.
<u>4</u>   Fill half of plastic sitz bowl with warm water, 94°-98° F (34°-37° C).
<u>6</u>   Dry area and reapply dressing or pad, if necessary.
<u>5</u>   Instruct client to open clamp of water bag to let warmer water into bowl.

2. Applying hot compresses

<u>4</u>   Wring out compress and apply to area.
<u>2</u>   Fill basin or container $1/2$ to $2/3$ full of water at 105°-115° F (40.5°-46.1° C).
<u>6</u>   Check client's skin every 10 minutes for danger signs.
<u>5</u>   Cover compress quickly with plastic wrap.
<u>1</u>   Place waterproof protector pad under the body part where compress is to be applied.
<u>3</u>   Put on gloves.

3. Applying elastic stocking

<u>3</u>   Place foot of stocking over client's toes, foot, and heel.
<u>1</u>   Put client in supine position.
<u>6</u>   Record what you have done.
<u>5</u>   Adjust stocking to fit smoothly without folds or wrinkles.
<u>2</u>   Turn stocking inside out, down to the heel.
<u>4</u>   Fit client's foot into heel and toe portion of stocking.

4. Assisting with transdermal disks

<u>2</u>   Have client remove and discard old disk into waste container.
<u>6</u>   Record what you have done.
<u>5</u>   Observe as client applies new disk to skin surface.
<u>4</u>   Ask client to select site for new disk.
<u>3</u>   Wash skin that had been covered by old disk.
<u>1</u>   Obtain materials.

Matching

1. F
2. G
3. A

ANSWERS

4. E
5. B
6. H
7. C
8. I
9. D
10. J

True or False

1. T
2. T
3. F A full glass of water or cool liquid is recommended.
4. T
5. T
6. T
7. T
8. F Clients should never double-up on a dose. They may take too much medication (an overdose). If a dose is omitted, notify your supervisor.
9. F Tell client not to take the medication until you have spoken with your supervisor.
10. T
11. T
12. F Unused medications should be discarded.
13. F Vaseline is not water-soluble. Use a water-soluble lubricant, such as K-Y jelly.
14. T
15. T
16. F Check every 10 minutes, more frequently for clients at great risk of burns.
17. T
18. F Keeping the legs under hot water causes blood vessels in legs to dilate. This decreases circulation to the perineal area.
19. T
20. T
21. F Home care aides NEVER regulate the flow of IV fluids. If there is a problem, call your supervisor.
22. T
23. T
24. T
25. F If elastic bandages are too tight they will shut off circulation. Apply firmly, but not too tightly.

What Needs To Be Corrected

1. Unplug and remove electric razor. Explain the risk of fire to client and family.
2. Use proper body mechanics; bend at knees. Elevate client's leg. Do procedure while client is in bed.

3. Properly tape dressing as shown in Figure 18-13 in text.
4. Bag of frozen peas should be covered.

CHAPTER 19

Caring for Older Adults

True or False

1. F Aging begins at birth.
2. F Incontinence is not a normal part of aging.
3. T
4. F One's personality usually does not change as aging progresses.
5. F Mental confusion is an abnormal condition.
6. F Do not try to change the subject. Listen and be patient.
7. F The need for home care will increase because of the increased numbers of older adults.
8. T
9. F The rate of aging depends on many factors including heredity, lifestyle, stresses in life, and one's occupation.
10. T
11. F It may take a little longer, but older adults can learn new things.
12. T
13. F The 85 and over age-group is the most rapidly growing age-group.
14. F Explain what you are going to do. Older adults understand what you say and need to know what will happen.
15. F Only 4.3% are cared for in institutions.

Normal Conditions of Aging

1. Difficulty adjusting to a dark room
   Have client wait a few minutes until the eyes have a chance to adjust to the darkness.
   Use a night light.
2. Forgets where eyeglasses were placed
   Encourage client to form the habit of placing eyeglasses in the same place.
   Encourage client to write reminders on a pad.
3. Dry skin
   Use soap sparingly.
   Apply moisturizers to skin after the bath.
4. Dry mouth
   Offer fluids frequently—1.5 to 2 qt (1500 to 2000 ml) daily.
   Give mouth care more frequently.

5. Complains of being cold
   Assist client to put on extra sweater; extra blanket.
   Caution client not to use heating pad or hot water bottle.
6. Occasional constipation
   Offer fluids frequently.
   Serve fruits, vegetables, and other high-fiber foods.
7. Shortness of breath with increased activity
   Provide frequent rest periods while assisting client with activities of daily living.
8. Anxious about changes in routine
   Do not change routines, if possible.
9. Urgent need to void
   For women, clothing should be easy to remove.
   Assist client to bathroom every 2 hours or less.
10. Feeling bloated
    Avoid serving gas-forming foods.
    Offer six to eight small meals per day.
11. Rapid heart beat when under stress
    Allow plenty of time to perform care procedures.
    Pace activities to avoid rushing.
12. Trouble adjusting to depths (going up and down stairs)
    Encourage client to use hand rails, if available.
    Provide support.
13. Trouble understanding what you are saying
    Speak slowly and clearly.
    Use short sentences.
14. Thick, hard toenails
    Do not cut or file.
    Notify supervisor—a podiatrist may be needed.
15. Unsteady balance when rising suddenly from a chair
    Have client count to 10 after rising and before proceeding to walk.
    Assist client to walk after counting to 10.

Situations

1. A. "You must be very upset. I don't know what I can do to help but I will talk to my supervisor about what you have told me."
      Encourage the daughter to contact your supervisor or the case manager.
   B. Leave the cases of beer under the bed.
   C. Notify your supervisor. Record what you said to the daughter; what you found; what you did about the cases of beer; and that you notified the supervisor.

2. A. Use nonverbal communication (hug, touch to hand) to show your concern.
   B. Report this situation to the supervisor after giving care to Magdalena.
   C. Record what her nephew said; the physical and emotional state of Magdalena; and that the supervisor was called.

D. "I can understand how upset you and your wife must be. Magdalena appears to be very upset, too. I was disturbed to see that Magdalena was so upset. I will contact my supervisor; perhaps we can find some solution to the problem."

3. A. Notify the supervisor.
   B. Help him to be properly groomed.
   C. Clean up the kitchen.
   D. Record all of the above.

CHAPTER 20

Caring for Mothers, Infants, and Children

Matching

1. C
2. E
3. I
4. G
5. J
6. D
7. A
8. F
9. H
10. B

Recognizing Normal and Abnormal Conditions in the Mother

1. ___ Complains of discomfort in the perineal area
2. ___ Weight loss of 19 lbs (8.6 kg) on the 10th day following delivery
3. _✗_ Three pads are used within 1 hour and contain a large number of blood clots
4. ___ Hemorrhoids in the anal area
5. _✗_ Cracked skin around the left nipple
6. _✗_ Elevated temperature—101° F (38.4° C) or higher
7. _✗_ Complains of tenderness in calf muscle of right leg
8. ___ Brownish colored lochia on the ninth day following delivery
9. ___ Mother says, "I feel so sad today, I just want to cry."
10. _✗_ Breasts are painful and hot to the touch
11. _✗_ Refuses to drink fluids because "My breasts will dry up faster."
12. _✗_ Vaginal discharge has a foul odor
13. ___ Lochia is scant and cream-colored on the 20th day following delivery
14. _✗_ Mother eats only skim milk, Jell-O, and dry crackers because she says, "I want to lose all the weight I gained. I hate being fat!"

15. ___ Tender breasts on the third day following delivery
16. _x_ No bowel movements for 5 days
17. _x_ Not interested in surroundings, withdrawn, and refuses to eat
18. _x_ Swelling and redness around the abdominal incision (cesarean birth)
19. ___ Complains of being exhausted on the second and third days following delivery
20. ___ Worries about being able to care for the infant properly

Situations

1. A. Put your arm around her and comfort her. Sit with her and listen to what she tells you. Offer to make her a cup of tea.
   B. Proceed to give her care as indicated in the care plan. Record the care given; what she said; and that your supervisor was notified.
   Report this incident to your supervisor.

2. A. Explain that Johnny's behavior is normal. He is jealous of all the attention that the new baby is getting.
   B. Report this to your supervisor.
   C. Help Yolanda to find ways to give Johny some special attention and let him know that he is still special to her.

True or False

1. T
2. F Infants sleep most of the day.
3. T
4. F Stools of breast-fed infants are pasty and mustard colored.
5. F Infants are burped halfway through a feeding as well as at the end.
6. T
7. T
8. T
9. F Newborns eat every 2 to 4 hours.
10. F Bottles warmed in the microwave may get too hot and burn the baby. Place bottle in pan of warm water.
11. T
12. T
13. F Children feel stress and experience strong reactions.
14. T
15. T

Observation

1. _x_ yellow skin
2. ___ bluish and cold hands and feet

3. ___ spitting up small amounts of feeding when burped
4. ___ crying and fussing every 3 hours
5. ___ wet diaper at every feeding
6. ___ sleeping most of the time
7. _x_ crying constantly; cannot be comforted
8. _x_ limp, hardly moves or cries
9. ___ has several yellow bowel movements a day
10. ___ cries during bath

ANSWERS

CHAPTER 21

Caring for Clients With Mental Illness

Crossword Puzzle

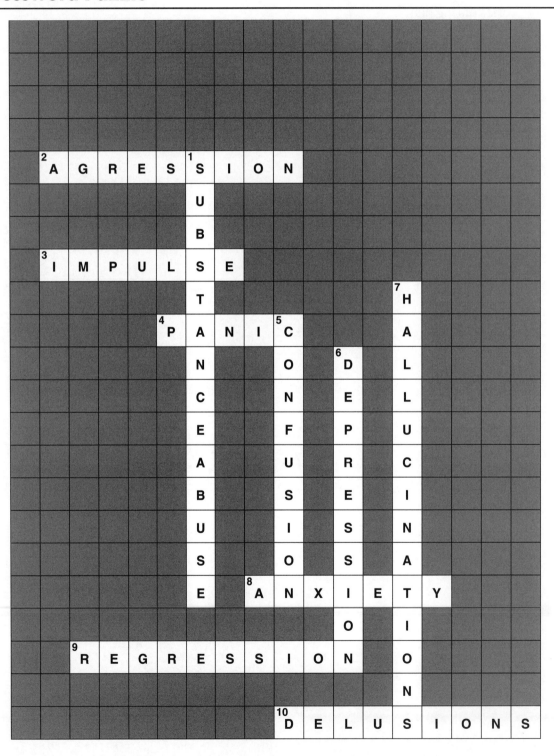

Situations

1. A. Offer finger foods and individual serving containers of fluid, if available, that can be eaten while she paces.
   B. Follow care plan schedule for toileting.
      Maintain fluid intake by offering fluids frequently.
   C. Assist with hygiene and grooming, as needed.

2. Assist him to dress correctly. Give directions in short, simple sentences. "Put on your socks. Put on your shoes. Tie your shoe laces."
   Encourage his wife to obtain an easy-to-read clock and calendar to help inform him about time and date.
   Place detergent and other potentially harmful substances and objects out of reach to provide a safe, secure environment.

3. A. Offer foods that cannot be tampered with, such as hard cooked eggs in their shells, with no cracks and individual unopened servings of food.
   B. Listen to what your client tells you. Tell him that you do not see or hear what he is seeing or hearing.
   C. Notify your supervisor immediately. Do not argue with the client.

4. A. Offer finger foods, small sandwiches, pieces of cheese, crackers, and other small foods rich in nutrition (raisins, grapes). Serve small, frequent feedings rather than three big meals. Report to your supervisor.
      Use a straw so client doesn't have to lift glass or cup. Put only a small amount into glass. Use very small glasses, but offer drinks frequently.
   B. Take to the bathroom according to schedule in care plan. Have client use commode if appropriate.
   C. Acknowledge his feelings by saying, "You seem very unhappy today."
   D. Report his comments to your supervisor. He may be considering suicide.

5. A. Watch client carefully. Try to find some diversions for her such as cards, checkers, reading to her, etc. Attach a bell to the door as a signal when it is opened. Take her out, when possible, to sit on the porch or walk in the neighborhood.
      Dress client in layers that take some time to remove.
   B. Keep a large robe handy, wrap around client, redress without any comment as to "good" or "bad" behavior.

6. Notify your supervisor.

7. A. Tell her, "No, thank you. I need to be alert to care for my client. I don't use anything like that."
   B. Notify your supervisor.

CHAPTER 22

Caring for Clients With Illnesses Requiring Home Care

Client Conditions

1. Wandering
   Approach client calmly and gradually guide him/her back, if wandering outside the home.
   Distract with offer of favorite snack or drink.
   Make sure client wears identification bracelet.

2. Fatigue
   Perform care activities when energy is at highest level, if possible. Allow plenty of time for client to perform activities of daily living. Do not rush. Provide frequent rest periods during bathing or dressing.

3. Difficulty swallowing
   Give thickened liquids, pureed or soft foods. Avoid foods that require a lot of chewing.
   Encourage client to use techniques taught by the occupational therapist.

4. Pain
   Use techniques listed in the care plan to help the client to tolerate pain (back rub, warm or cool applications to the area).
   Bring pain medication to client on time, according to the care plan.

5. Paralysis or weakness on right side of the body
   Do not pull on the right arm or leg when lifting or moving the client.
   Assist client to use assistive devices (soap on a rope) as directed by the occupational or physical therapist.

6. Diarrhea
   Keep anal area clean and dry. Wear disposable gloves when cleaning the client's skin and anal area. Keep bedpan or commode handy for easy use.
   Encourage client to drink lots of fluids, according to the care plan.

7. Difficulty breathing
   Place in Fowler's position or use two or more pillows to support the upper back.
   Use energy-saving techniques, such as providing frequent rest periods during bathing and dressing. Do not rush the client.

8. Sores in the mouth
   Be gentle when giving mouth care. Wear disposable gloves. Use normal saline solution instead of alcohol-based mouth wash.
   Use soft bristled tooth brush or foam swab.

Situations

1. A. Lock doors to dangerous areas (basement, garage).
   Remove matches, lighter fluid, and other flammable liquids.
   Remove control knobs from the stove.
   Place plastic bags out of reach.
   Remove food-shaped kitchen magnets, coins, and other small objects.
   B. Try to find the location of her favorite hiding places (under the bed or pillows). Then check these places first. Offer to help her to find the eyeglasses. Remain calm.
   C. Make name tags for each family member. Include name and title (daughter, son-in-law, granddaughter) to help the mother to remember. Have family members wear the name tags. You may wish to make tags for other relatives and friends.
   D. Be alert for signs that your mother needs to use the bathroom, such as restlessness. Plan a routine to take her to the toilet before accidents occur. Put a sign that says "Bathroom" and a picture of a toilet on the bathroom door.
   E. Support groups help caregivers in a variety of ways. These include providing the chance to share caregiving experiences with others in similar situations and discussing ways of handling problems. You may find that participating in the support group will give you encouragement and strength to continue to care for your mother.

2. A. Place chair in the bathroom so he can sit by the sink. Place toilet articles within easy reach for Mr. Yancy to use.
   B. Do not wash off the markings. Do not wash the skin inside the markings.
   C. Select foods that do not require a lot of energy to chew. Offer small, frequent meals. Prepare foods that Mr. Yancy enjoys eating. Prepare foods (pour coffee, butter bread) so that Mr. Yancy can use his energy to eat, not for these activities.
   D. Changes in the type or frequency of pain
   Signs of infection
   Bruising or bleeding
   Problems with eating, swallowing, or drinking

3. A. 1. Wear disposable gloves while giving him mouth care because of risk of contact with blood from bleeding gums.
   2. Wear disposable gloves when cleaning his skin of fecal material following a bout with diarrhea because of risk of contact with blood in the fecal material.
   3. Prepare bleach solution daily. Fresh solution is needed to maintain its effectiveness. Use for cleaning up spill of body fluids and soaking fecal-stained clothing and bed linens. Bleach solution destroys the human immunodeficiency virus.
   4. Wear disposable gloves whenever there is risk of coming in contact with bloody fluids to protect yourself from infection.
   5. Avoid splashing when disposing of contents of bedpan and urinal to prevent spread of organisms. Wear mask and goggles, if necessary.
   B. Carefully clean and dry the areas thoroughly. Record location and size of each reddened area and report to your supervisor immediately.
   C. Prepare and store foods properly.
   Wash fresh fruits and vegetables thoroughly.

Refrigerate leftovers immediately.

    D. No. I've been trained to take special precautions when caring for Fernando to protect myself and to protect him from infections from others. I'm not very brave, I'm just doing my job.

    E. Do not be afraid to touch and hug your brother. Showing affection is very important.

4. A. Report to supervisor.
    B. Tell her to hold a pillow next to the incision and press it in while she coughs.
    C. Notify your supervisor.

5. A. Remove any object that may cause client to fall. Walk next to her to provide support and assistance as needed.
    B. Puree foods as needed and follow care plan for thickening foods, if necessary. Remind client about swallowing as taught by speech therapist.
    C. Try to anticipate her needs and ask questions that can be answered with a "yes" or "no" instead of a complicated answer. Use pictures, if available.
    D. Be patient with her and point out how well she is doing and how much she has improved.

6. Notify the supervisor immediately.

True or False

1. T
2. T
3. T
4. T
5. F Cancer treatments often cause many side effects including loss of hair, sores in the mouth, and bleeding gums.
6. F Parkinson's disease is a chronic illness affecting people in late middle age and older adulthood.
7. T
8. T
9. F Reasoning will not help an Alzheimer's client understand what is happening; it may confuse and agitate the client.
10. T
11. T
12. T
13. T
14. F Standard (Universal) precautions are used with all clients.
15. T
16. T
17. F Clients may shower with a cast (according to the care plan), provided the cast is wrapped in plastic and protected from water. Never soak a cast or allow a cast to become soaked.
18. F Immediately report these symptoms to your supervisor. They indicate a problem with nerve and blood supply to the casted part.
19. T
20. T
21. F Sterile dressings are changed by the nurse.

22. F "Phantom limb pain" is real pain, not imagined.
23. T
24. F Too much food is overwhelming. Offer small frequent feedings.
25. T

CHAPTER 23

Caring for the Dying Client

Completion

1. Emotional responses to dying are <u>denial</u>, <u>anger</u>, <u>bargaining</u>, <u>depression</u>, and <u>acceptance</u>.
2. A final illness from which a client is not expected to recover is called a <u>terminal</u> illness or an <u>end-stage</u> disease.
3. Living will and durable power of attorney are examples of <u>advance medical directives</u>.
4. A program that cares for the dying client and his or her caregivers is <u>hospice</u>.
5. Two signs of approaching death are <u>slowed circulation</u> and <u>cold hands and feet</u>.
   unconsciousness
   difficulty breathing
   any other symptoms listed in the text
6. The last sense to leave the body is <u>hearing</u>.
7. Care given after death is called <u>postmortem</u> care.

Situations

1. Ask Mr. Toomey why he is asking you about his death. Listen to what he says. If he doesn't understand what is happening, speak with your supervisor.
2. Discuss the situation with your supervisor to determine if your client is depressed about dying and is withdrawing in preparation for death. If so, your supervisor will explain to caregivers.
3. Even though the hope of a "miracle cure" may seem totally unrealistic, members of the health-care team share that hope with clients and caregivers. If denial is present, recognize that both client and caregivers need that denial to cope with the emotional stresses of the illness.
4. Recognize Josephine's anger by saying, "Josephine, you seem to be very angry today." Then ask her to tell you about her feelings by saying, "Can you tell me how you're feeling?"
5. It's OK to be sad when your client dies. Call your agency and speak to your supervisor about these feelings. It helps to talk about your emotions.
6. Notify your supervisor to make sure the agency knows about these religious practices. Follow agency policy regarding the pronouncement of death. Respect caregiver's religious practices.
7. Inform the family that hearing is the last sense to leave the body of a dying person. They should say their "goodbyes."

CHAPTER 24

Emergencies

Completion

1. The emergency telephone number to call in my area is _____.
2. The Poison Control Center's telephone number in my area is _____.
3. The four Cs of Emergency Care are <u>caution—do not put yourself in danger, check—your local emergency number, call—your local emergency number,</u> and <u>care—for the victim until help arrives.</u>
4. First aid situations that increase the home care aide's risk for infection are <u>bleeding victim, wound is weeping fluid,</u> and <u>wound was caused by an animal bite.</u>
5. The four signs of a medical emergency that require immediate action are <u>unconsciousness, no breathing, no pulse,</u> and <u>severe bleeding.</u>

Situations (A)

1. A. Use barrier to protect yourself from blood (e.g., plastic bag, plastic wrap, disposable gloves).
   B. Apply sterile or clean dressing over the wound.
   C. Apply direct pressure over the wound.
   D. Apply bandage snugly over the dressing to keep it in place.

2. A. Assist victim into position with head lower than the legs. If injury to back, head, or neck is suspected, keep victim flat.
   B. Loosen any tight clothing to make breathing easier.
   C. Maintain body temperature (cover with sweater, blanket).
   D. Reassure victim that help is coming.

3. A. Run cool tap water over the burned area to cool the skin and reduce the burning process.
   B. Cover the burn, using a dry, sterile dressing or dry, clean cloth to prevent infection.
   C. Apply loose bandage to keep dressing in place.
   D. Do not break the blisters.

4. A. Help her to lie on the floor.
   B. Remove any furniture or other objects that the victim might strike against during uncontrolled body movements.
   C. Protect her from injury.
   D. Do not restrict her movements or place anything in her mouth.

5. A. Stand behind victim and wrap your arms around the victim's waist.
   B. Make a fist with one hand and place the thumb side against the middle of the victim's abdomen, just above the navel and below the rib cage.

C. Grab your fist with your other hand and give quick, inward, and upward thrusts into the abdomen.

D. Repeat thrusts until the object is forced out.

6. A. Do not move the client and ask her not to move.

B. Maintain body temperature.

C. Remain with the client.

D. Reassure and comfort the client.

7. A. Have him sit down immediately.

B. Loosen tight clothing.

C. Reassure him that help is on the way.

D. Help him to remain calm.

Situations (B)

1. Stop her, place her on the ground, then roll her to smother the flames.

2. A. Adhesive tape

B. Gauze pads

C. Scissors

D. Adhesive bandages

E. Hand cleaner

F. Disposable gloves

3. A. Remove the container of toilet bowl cleaner from Louisa.

B. Take her out of the bathroom.
Call the Poison Control Center and report the name of the toilet bowl cleaner and the time you found Louisa drinking the fluid.

4. A. Your client's name or the victim's name

B. The type of emergency

C. Where and when it happened

D. What first aid was given and who was called

CHAPTER 25

Getting a Job and Keeping It
Crossword Puzzle

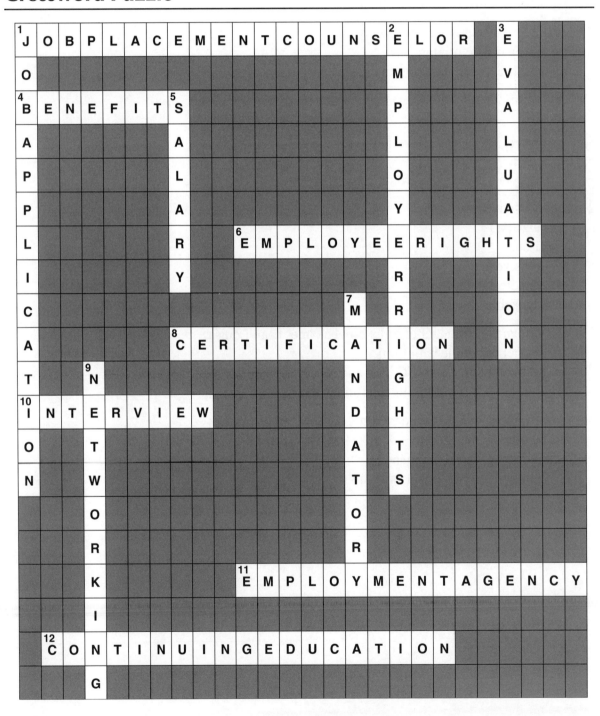

Want Ad

1. A. experience
   B. preferred
   C. certification
   D. required
   E. excellent
   F. reimbursement

2. A. You are reimbursed for travel while on the job.
   B. Work can be Monday through Friday and weekends, too.
   C. Living in the client's home while providing care.
   D. Benefits mean medical, dental, and life insurance; paid vacation; sick days, etc.

3. A. Having a paper and pen handy to take notes
   B. Having any general questions ready to ask

The Job Interview

1. You should arrive no later than 1:20 PM.
2. Sample application form (Workbook Figure 25-1: Answers will vary)
3. Ask her to explain the travel requirements and uniforms.
4. A.
     1. Give care according to the care plan.
     2. Perform duties correctly.
   B.
     1. Use correct forms.
     2. Record client care and billable time.
   C.
     1. Practice safety awareness at all times.
     2. Use standard (universal) precautions when needed.
   D.
     1. Accept constructive criticism given by the supervisor.
     2. Follow suggestions for improving job performance.
5. A.
     1. Provide necessary equipment and supplies to protect me from possible infection.
     2. Remove me from situations in the home where there is danger.
   B.
     1. Provide payment according to an agreed-upon rate and according to pay scale.
     2. Provide correct amount of money for the time I worked.
   C.
     1. Regularly supervise me on the job.
     2. Respond promptly when I contact the agency to report abnormal conditions of my client.

D.
1. Inform me of the results of the evaluations.
2. If my evaluation is not satisfactory, inform me about what will happen if my performance does not improve.

6. A. <u>No</u>
   B. <u>Yes</u>
   C. <u>No</u>
   D. <u>No</u>
   E. <u>Yes</u>
   F. <u>No</u>
   G. <u>Yes</u>
   H. <u>Yes</u>
   I. <u>No</u>

Skills Competency Checklists

Procedure 10-1.   Feeding the Client

Name: _____

	S	UN

1. Explained procedure to client.
2. Washed hands.
3. Obtained necessary materials.
4. Prepared client for mealtime:
   Offered to assist with toileting
   Offered to assist client to wash hands
   Positioned client to sit up in bed/chair
   Placed table or bed tray over client's lap
5. Draped napkin across client's chest and under chin.
6. Served food on tray, if needed.
7. Sat near client.
8. Explained what is being served.
9. Cut food, buttered bread, and prepared liquids as needed.
10. Asked client what he/she would like to eat first
11. Encouraged self-feeding, if appropriate.
12. Fed client (one bite at a time—one-half spoon full).
    Allowed time to chew and swallow.
13. Alternated solids and liquids; used straw if needed.
14. Talked with client and offered praise for eating.
15. Wiped client's mouth and removed tray (if used) when
    client finished.
16. Washed client's face and hands. Removed napkin or bib.
17. Offered oral hygiene.
18. Made sure client was safe and comfortable.
19. Recorded in care record percent of food consumed.
20. Washed hands.
21. Washed dishes and utensils used for meal.
22. Cleaned and straightened kitchen.

Comments:

Evaluator's Signature: _____
Date: _____

Procedure 11-1.   Hand Washing

Name: _____

	S	UN
1. Collected all materials at the sink.	___	___
2. Removed watch (or pushed up forearm 4-5 inches) and rings.	___	___
3. Stood back from sink to keep clothing from becoming wet.	___	___
4. Turned on faucet and adjusted water to comfortable temperature.	___	___
5. Wet hands and wrists completely. Kept fingers and hands below elbows.	___	___
6. Applied soap to hands.	___	___
7. Lathered hands well by rubbing palms together. Spread lather over hands and wrists, under nails, and between fingers.	___	___
8. Used rotating and rubbing motion for 30 seconds.	___	___
a. Vigorously rubbed one hand against the other and around wrist. Repeated with the other hand and wrist.	___	___
b. Washed between fingers by interlacing them.		
c. Rubbed fingernails against the palms of hands.	___	___
9. Washed at least two inches above the wrist.	___	___
10. Rinsed well, one hand at a time. Rinsed from 2 inches above the wrist and kept hands and fingers below the elbows.	___	___
11. Dried hands and wrists with paper towels.		
12. Dropped the used paper towels into wastebasket.	___	___
13. Turned off faucets using another dry paper towel.	___	___
14. Discarded towel.	___	___
15. Applied hand lotion, if desired.	___	___

Comments:

Evaluator's Signature: _____
Date: _____

Procedure 11-2.   Applying Gloves and Removing Contaminated Gloves

Name: _____

	S	UN
APPLYING GLOVES		
1. Washed hands.	____	____
2. Dried hands thoroughly.	____	____
3. Inspected gloves for tears or perforations.	____	____
4. Put gloves on when ready to begin client care.	____	____

	S	UN
REMOVING CONTAMINATED GLOVES (BOTH HANDS STILL GLOVED)		
1. Used right hand to grasp glove on left hand. Grasped outer surface of glove just below the wrist cuff.	____	____
2. Pulled left glove downward until it was off and turned inside out.	____	____
3. Continued to hold left glove in right hand. Gathered up glove in right hand.	____	____
4. Inserted two fingers of left hand inside cuff of right glove. Did not touch outside of glove with bare hand.	____	____
5. Pulled right glove down and inside out and completely over left glove.	____	____
6. Deposited both gloves in proper container.	____	____
7. Washed hands.	____	____

Comments:

Evaluator's Signature: _____
Date: _____

Procedure 11-3. Disinfecting Using Wet Heat

Name: _____

	S	UN
1. Washed hands.	___	___
2. Placed items in pot so that all surfaces were in contact with water.	___	___
3. Covered items with water. Provided some space at top of pot for steam to escape.	___	___
4. Placed lid on top of pot.	___	___
5. Placed covered pot on stove or other source of heat. Checked to see that bottom of pot was in full contact with heat source.	___	___
6. Turned pot handle(s) to the side(s).	___	___
7. Turned on heat and brought water to a boil.	___	___
8. Boiled for 20 minutes without lifting pot lid.	___	___
9. Turned off heat.	___	___
10. Allowed water and contents to cool.	___	___
11. Removed cover with potholder.	___	___
12. Removed disinfected items. Placed on clean towel to air dry. Stored properly.	___	___
13. Washed, dried, and returned disinfecting supplies to appropriate location.	___	___
14. Washed hands.	___	___

Comments:

Evaluator's Signature: _____

Date: _____

Procedure 11-4.   Disinfecting Using Dry Heat

Name: _____

	S	UN
1. Washed hands.	___	___
2. Placed cloth-wrapped dressings in flat pan.	___	___
3. Placed flat pan in oven.	___	___
4. Pre-heated oven to 350° F (180°C).	___	___
5. Allowed items to bake for 1 hour without opening oven.	___	___
6. Turned off oven and allowed items to cool.	___	___
7. Removed flat pan using pot holder.	___	___
8. Unwrapped cloth carefully without touching dressings.	___	___
9. Returned items to appropriate location.	___	___
10. Washed hands.	___	___

Comments:

Evaluator's Signature: _____

Date: _____

Procedure 11-5.   Making Bleach Solution

Name: _____

	S	UN
1. Washed hands.	___	___
2. Put on rubber utility gloves.	___	___
3. Measured 5 cups (1200 ml) of water; poured into container.	___	___
4. Measured 1/2 cup (120 ml) of household bleach; added to container.	___	___
5. Placed cap on container and shook to mix solution.	___	___
6. Prepared label, "Bleach Solution 1:10," dated, and applied to container.	___	___
7. Stored in closed cabinet, out of reach of children, and away from foods. Returned materials to appropriate location.	___	___
8. Removed and rinsed gloves. Hung them up to dry.	___	___
9. Washed hands.	___	___

Comments:

Evaluator's Signature: _____

Date: _____

Procedure 11-6.   Making Vinegar Solution

Name: _____

	S	UN
1. Washed hands.	___	___
2. Measured 3 cups (720 ml) of water, and poured into container.	___	___
3. Measured 1 cup (240 ml) of white vinegar; and added to container.	___	___
4. Placed cap on container and shook to mix solution.	___	___
5. Prepared label, "Vinegar Solution 1:3," dated, and applied to container.	___	___
6. Stored in closed cabinet, out of reach of children, and away from food. Returned materials to appropriate location.	___	___
7. Washed hands.	___	___

Comments:

Evaluator's Signature: _____
Date: _____

Procedure 11-7.   Disinfecting With Household Solutions

Name: _____

	S	UN
1. Washed hands.	___	___
2. Put on rubber utility gloves.	___	___
3. Washed items with detergent.	___	___
4. Rinsed items with warm water.	___	___
5. Poured solution into plastic pan.	___	___
6. Submerged washed items in solution for 10 minutes.	___	___
7. Removed items.	___	___
8. Rinsed well with hot water.	___	___
9. Laid items on paper towel to dry or hung on towel rack or shower rail to dry.	___	___
10. Cleaned area and returned materials to appropriate location.	___	___
11. Removed and rinsed gloves. Hung up to dry.	___	___
12. Washed hands.	___	___

Comments:

Evaluator's Signature: _____

Date: _____

Procedure 11-8.   Applying a Mask and Removing a Contaminated Mask

Name: _____

APPLYING MASK	S	UN
1. Washed hands.	___	___
2. Picked up mask by top strings (or upper elastic band).	___	___
3. Positioned mask over nose and mouth with top strings over ears. Tied strings behind head (or positioned elastic band over ears and high up on head).	___	___
4. Tied lower strings (or positioned lower elastic band low on back of head, under ears).	___	___

REMOVING CONTAMINATED MASK	S	UN
1. Washed hands.	___	___
2. Untied lower strings of mask (or pulled lower elastic band up to top of head).	___	___
3. Untied upper strings and removed mask while still holding strings (or lifted both elastic bands over head and removed mask).	___	___
4. Discarded mask in proper container.	___	___
5. Washed hands.	___	___

Comments:

Evaluator's Signature: _____
Date: _____

Procedure 11-9.   Applying a Gown and Removing a Contaminated Gown

Name: _____

APPLYING GOWN	S	UN
1. Washed hands.	____	____
2. Inserted arms into sleeves of gown with opening in the back.	____	____
3. Tied the neck strings (or closed Velcro strips).	____	____
4. Closed the back opening by overlapping one side of gown over the other.	____	____
5. Tied gown at waist (or closed Velcro strips).	____	____

REMOVING CONTAMINATED GOWN	S	UN
1. Untied waist strings.	____	____
2. Untied neck strings.	____	____
3. Pulled gown down from the shoulder with neck ties.	____	____
4. Leaned forward, turned the gown inside out while removing it. Did not touch the outside of the gown.	____	____
5. Kept one hand inside the sleeve of the gown, used it to pull off the other sleeve. Did the same on the other side.	____	____
6. Rolled up the gown into a ball. Kept contaminated area inside.	____	____
7. Discarded into proper container.	____	____
8. Washed hands.	____	____

Comments:

Evaluator's Signature: _____

Date: _____

Procedure 11-10.   Double Bagging

Name: _____

	S	UN
1. Have helper positioned outside of client's door with a "clean bag." If alone, placed clean bag in doorway.	____	____
2. Washed hands.	____	____
3. Applied gown and gloves.	____	____
4. Entered room, took in "dirty" bag.	____	____
5. Placed contaminated materials in "dirty" bag.	____	____
6. Asked person with "clean" bag to open it for insertion of second (dirty) bag. Helper sealed "clean" bag. If alone, placed "dirty" bag in "clean" bag without sealing it until hands are clean.	____	____
7. Removed gloves and gown. Discarded in proper container.	____	____
8. Washed hands. If alone, sealed "clean" bag containing "dirty" bag.	____	____
9. Disposed of double-bagged material properly	____	____

Comments:

Evaluator's Signature: _____

Date: _____

Procedure 12-1.   Raising Client's Head and Shoulders

Name: _____

	S	UN
1. Explained procedure to client.	____	____
2. Washed hands.	____	____
3. Provided privacy.	____	____
4. Raised bed to convenient working height.*	____	____
5. Locked wheels on bed, or pushed bed against wall if there are no brakes.*	____	____
6. Lowered rail on side of bed on side where aide is working.*	____	____
7. Lowered head of bed, removed pillows. Folded back top sheet.	____	____
8. Stood facing bed with feet about 12 inches apart.	____	____
9. Asked client to place near arm under aide's near arm and shoulder. (Client's hand should reach aide's shoulder.)	____	____
10. Placed aide's near arm under client's arm and shoulder. (Aide's hand should reach client's shoulder.)	____	____
11. Slipped farthest arm under client's neck and shoulders.	____	____
12. On count of "3", aide shifted weight from foot nearest head of the bed to the other foot. At the same time, client was rocked to a semi-sitting position.	____	____
13. Supported client with arm locked under client's shoulder; pillows removed or readjusted using other arm.	____	____
14. Assisted client to lie back on bed using locked arms and supporting neck and shoulders as before.	____	____
15. Made sure client was safe and comfortable. Replaced top sheet.	____	____
16. Placed bed in lowest position. (Raised side rail, if indicated.)*	____	____
17. Washed hands.	____	____

Comments:

Evaluator's Signature: _____
Date: _____

*Will not apply if hospital bed is not used.

Procedure 12-2.   Moving Client to Side of Bed

Name: _____

		S	UN
1.	Explained procedure to client.	___	___
2.	Washed hands.	___	___
3.	Provided privacy.	___	___
4.	Raised bed to convenient working height.*	___	___
5.	Locked wheels on bed, or pushed bed against wall if there are no brakes.*	___	___
6.	Lowered rail on side of bed on side where aide is working.*	___	___
7.	Folded back top sheet.	___	___
8.	Stood facing bed with feet about 12 inches apart, one foot in front of the other. Shifted weight from front to rear foot as each move was performed.	___	___
9.	Slipped one arm under client and reached across to the opposite shoulder. Placed other arm under middle of client's back.	___	___
10.	On count of "3", aide rocked back and shifted upper segment of client's body to edge of bed.	___	___
11.	Placed arms under client's waist and buttocks. Moved to edge of bed in same manner.	___	___
12.	Placed arms under client's thighs and lower legs. Moved to edge of bed in same manner.	___	___
13.	Made sure client is in good body alignment. Replaced top sheet.	___	___
14.	Placed bed in lowest position. (Raised side rail if indicated.)*	___	___
15.	Made sure client was safe and comfortable. Replaced top sheet.	___	___
16.	Placed bed in lowest position. (Raised side rail, if indicated.)*	___	___
17.	Washed hands.	___	___

Comments:

Evaluator's Signature: _____
Date: _____

*Will not apply if hospital bed is not used.

Procedure 12-3.   Moving Up in Bed When Client Can Help

Name: _____

	S	UN
1. Explained procedure to client.	___	___
2. Washed hands.	___	___
3. Provided privacy.	___	___
4. Raised bed to convenient working height.*	___	___
5. Locked wheels on bed, or pushed bed against wall if there are no brakes.*	___	___
6. Lowered rail on side of bed on side where aide is working.*	___	___
7. Folded back top sheet. Lowered client's head; removed pillows.	___	___
8. Propped one pillow against headboard to protect client's head.	___	___
9. Stood facing head of bed, knees bent, feet about 12 inches apart.	___	___
10. Slipped one arm under client's shoulders; the other under client's thighs.	___	___
11. Instructed client to bend his or her knees and to firmly place feet against mattress. Gave signal to client to push with hands and feet to assist with move up in bed.	___	___
12. Helped client move toward head of bed by shifting body weight from back leg to front leg.	___	___
13. Used several small, upward moves rather than one large move to reach head of bed.	___	___
14. Made sure client is in good body alignment. Replaced top sheet and pillows.	___	___
15. Placed bed in lowest position. (Raised side rail if indicated.)*	___	___
16. Washed hands.	___	___

Comments:

Evaluator's Signature: _____
Date: _____

*Will not apply if hospital bed is not used.

Procedure 12-4.　Moving Up in Bed When Client Cannot Help

Name: _____

	S	UN
1. Explained procedure to client.	___	___
2. Washed hands.	___	___
3. Provided privacy.	___	___
4. Raised bed to convenient working height.*	___	___
5. Locked wheels on bed, or pushed bed against wall if there are no brakes.*	___	___
6. Lowered rail on side of bed on side where aide is working.*	___	___
7. Folded back top sheet. Lowered client's head; removed pillows.	___	___
8. Propped one pillow against headboard to protect client's head.	___	___
9. Made sure turning sheet was in position under client's body.	___	___
10. **One person:**		
a. Kept side rails up.*	___	___
b. Stood at head of bed with feet about 12 inches apart, one foot in front of the other, and faced the bed.	___	___
c. Rolled top of turning sheet toward client's head.	___	___
d. Firmly grasped top of turning sheet with both hands.	___	___
e. Used good body mechanics—bent knees and hips, kept back straight.	___	___
f. On count of "3", shifted weight from front leg to back leg, pulled turning sheet and client up toward head of bed.	___	___
11. **Two persons:**		
a. Lowered both side rails.*	___	___
b. Aide took place at one side of bed with feet 12 inches apart, one foot in front of the other and faced head of bed. (Other person or aide did same.)	___	___
c. Sides of turning sheet were rolled close to client's body.	___	___
d. Turning sheet edges were firmly grasped with both hands.	___	___
e. Used good body mechanics—bent knees and hips, kept back straight.	___	___
f. On count of "3", aide and helper shifted body weight from rear leg to front leg, lifted turning sheet and moved client toward head of bed.	___	___
12. Checked lower sheets for wrinkles; smoothed, if necessary.	___	___
13. Made sure client was in good body alignment. Replaced top sheet and pillows.	___	___
14. Placed bed in lowest position. (Raised side rail, if indicated.)*	___	___
15. Washed hands.	___	___

Comments:

Evaluator's Signature: _____
Date: _____

*Will not apply if hospital bed is not used.

Procedure 12-5.   Positioning Client in Supine (Back-lying) Position

Name: _____

	S	UN
1. Explained procedure to client.	____	____
2. Washed hands.	____	____
3. Provided privacy.	____	____
4. Raised bed to convenient working height.*	____	____
5. Locked wheels on bed, or pushed bed against wall if there are no brakes.*	____	____
6. Lowered rail on side of bed on side where aide is working.*	____	____
7. Folded back top sheet. Positioned client on back.	____	____
8. Adjusted pillows properly:	____	____
a. Small pillow under head and shoulders	____	____
b. Supported arms and hands with pillows	____	____
c. Small pillow or folded towel placed under small of back (if supervisor has so instructed).	____	____
9. Positioned other devices, such as footboard, trochanter rolls, bed cradle, as indicated in care plan.	____	____
10. Made sure client is in proper body alignment. Replaced top sheet.	____	____
11. Placed bed in lowest position. (Raised side rail, if indicated.)*	____	____
12. Washed hands.	____	____
13. Recorded what was done.	____	____

Comments:

Evaluator's Signature: _____
Date: _____

*Will not apply if hospital bed is not used.

Procedure 12-6.   Positioning Client in Fowler's (Semi-sitting) Position

Name: _____

	S	UN
1. Explained procedure to client.	___	___
2. Washed hands.	___	___
3. Provided privacy.	___	___
4. Raised bed to convenient working height.*	___	___
5. Locked wheels on bed, or pushed bed against wall if there are no brakes.*	___	___
6. Lowered rail on side of bed on side where aide is working.*	___	___
7. Folded back top sheet. Positioned client on back.	___	___
8. Raised head of bed to 45-degree angle. If bed was not adjustable, used other devices to position client.	___	___
9. Adjusted pillows properly:	___	___
a. Small pillow under head and shoulders	___	___
b. Supported arms and hands with pillows	___	___
10. Positioned other devices, such as footboard, trochanter rolls, bed cradle, as indicated in care plan.	___	___
11. Made sure client is in proper body alignment. Replaced top sheet.	___	___
12. Placed bed in lowest position. (Raised side rail, if indicated.)*	___	___
13. Washed hands.	___	___
14. Recorded what was done.	___	___

Comments:

Evaluator's Signature: _____
Date: _____

*Will not apply if hospital bed is not used.

Procedure 12-7.   Positioning Client in Lateral (Side-lying) Position

Name: _____

	S	UN
1. Explained procedure to client.	___	___
2. Washed hands.	___	___
3. Provided privacy.	___	___
4. Raised bed to convenient working height.*	___	___
5. Locked wheels on bed, or pushed bed against wall if there are no brakes.*	___	___
6. Lowered rail on side of bed on side where aide is working.*	___	___
7. Lowered client's head; removed pillows. Folded back top sheet.	___	___
8. Asked client to move to side of bed nearest aide. Assisted client as needed.	___	___
9. Raised side rail.*	___	___
10. Went to other side of bed and lowered side rail.*	___	___
11. Placed one hand around client's farthest shoulder and the other hand around client's farthest hip. Rolled client toward aide and turned client on side facing toward center of bed. Bent client's upper leg and both arms.	___	___
12. Adjusted pillows properly:		
a. Small pillow under head and neck	___	___
b. Supported upper arm and leg on pillows	___	___
c. Folded towel placed along back to maintain side-lying position (optional).	___	___
13. Positioned other devices as indicated in the care plan.	___	___
14. Made sure client is in good body alignment. Replaced top sheet.	___	___
15. Placed bed in lowest position. (Raised side rail, if indicated.)*	___	___
16. Washed hands.	___	___
17. Recorded what was done.	___	___

Comments:

Evaluator's Signature: _____

Date: _____

*Will not apply if hospital bed is not used.

Procedure 12-8.   Positioning Client in Sims' Position

Name: _____

	S	**UN**
1. Explained procedure to client.	___	___
2. Washed hands.	___	___
3. Provided privacy.	___	___
4. Raised bed to convenient working height.*	___	___
5. Locked wheels on bed, or pushed bed against wall if there are no brakes.*	___	___
6. Lowered rail on side of bed on side where aide is working.*	___	___
7. Lowered client's head; removed pillows. Folded back top sheet.	___	___
8. Asked client to move to side of bed nearest aide. Assisted client as needed.	___	___
9. Raised side rail.*	___	___
10. Went to other side of bed and lowered side rail.*	___	___
11. Placed one hand around client's farthest shoulder and the other hand around client's farthest hip. Rolled client toward aide and turned client on side facing toward center of bed. Positioned upper leg so it did not rest on lower leg. (Lower arm should be behind client.)	___	___
12. Adjusted pillows properly:	___	___
a. Small pillow under head and neck.	___	___
b. Supported upper arm and leg on pillows.	___	___
13. Positioned other devices as indicated in the care plan.	___	___
14. Made sure client is in good body alignment. Replaced top sheet.	___	___
15. Placed bed in lowest position. (Raised side rail, if indicated.)*	___	___
16. Washed hands.	___	___
17. Recorded what was done. Reported any unusual conditions to supervisor.	___	___

Comments:

Evaluator's Signature: _____
Date: _____

*Will not apply if hospital bed is not used.

Procedure 12-9.   Positioning Client in Prone (Abdominal) Position

Name: _____

	S	UN
1. Explained procedure to client.		
2. Washed hands.		
3. Provided privacy.		
4. Raised bed to convenient working height.*		
5. Locked wheels on bed, or pushed bed against wall if there are no brakes.*		
6. Lowered rail on side of bed on side where aide is working.*		
7. Lowered client's head; removed pillows. Folded back top sheet.		
8. Asked client to move to side of bed nearest aide. Assisted client as needed.		
9. Raised side rail.*		
10. Went to other side of bed and lowered side rail.*		
11. Placed one hand around client's farthest shoulder and the other hand around client's farthest hip. Rolled client toward aide and turned client on side, then onto abdomen. Turned client's head to side. Arms are flexed on each side of head.		
12. Adjusted pillows properly:		
a. Small pillow under head and neck.		
b. Optional small pillow under abdomen.		
c. Pillow placed under lower legs to relieve pressure on toes. Client may be positioned so that toes hang over mattress.		
13. Made sure client is in good body alignment. Replaced top sheet.		
15. Placed bed in lowest position. (Raised side rail, if indicated.)*		
16. Washed hands.		
17. Recorded what was done. Reported any unusual conditions to supervisor.		

Comments:

Evaluator's Signature: _____
Date: _____

*Will not apply if hospital bed is not used.

Procedure 12-10.   Assisting Client to Sit on Side of Bed

Name: _____

	S	UN
1. Explained procedure to client.	____	____
2. Washed hands.	____	____
3. Obtained necessary materials.	____	____
4. Provided privacy.	____	____
5. Raised bed to convenient working height.*	____	____
6. Locked wheels on bed, or pushed bed against wall if there are not brakes.*	____	____
7. Lowered rail on side of bed on side where aide is working.*	____	____
8. Folded back top bedding.	____	____
9. Stood as close to side of bed as possible (legs touching side of bed); and was level with client	____	____
10. Positioned feet apart, with one foot staggered. Bent hips and knees.	____	____
11. Asked client to move to side of bed nearest aide. Assisted client as needed.	____	____
12. Put up side rail and raised head of bed.*	____	____
13. Placed client in Fowler's position without pillows.	____	____
14. Lowered bed and put side rail down.*	____	____
15. Placed one arm around the shoulder area and the other arm under client's knees.	____	____
16. On count of "3", shifted weight to back leg, and slowly swung client's legs over edge of bed while pulling shoulders to sitting position.	____	____
17. Placed bed in lowest position so client's feet are touching the floor.*	____	____
18. Remained facing client with both hands supporting shoulders until client was stable.	____	____
19. Assisted client to put on robe and footwear. Applied transfer or gait belt, if needed for transfer.	____	____
20. Placed back of chair next to bed, facing client. Had client hold back of chair to keep balance, if needed.	____	____
21. Remained with client.	____	____
22. Reversed procedure to return client to Fowler's position.	____	____
23. Washed hands.	____	____
24. Recorded client's reaction to procedure, amount of time spent sitting on side of bed, and any other observations.	____	____

Comments:

Evaluator's Signature: _____
Date: _____

*Will not apply if hospital bed is not used.

Procedure 12-11.   Transferring Client From Bed to Chair/Wheelchair—Standing Transfer

Name: _____

	S	UN
1. Explained procedure to client.	___	___
2. Washed hands.	___	___
3. Obtained necessary materials.	___	___
4. Provided privacy.	___	___
5. Placed chair parallel to bed and on client's strong side.	___	___
6. If wheelchair was used, locked brakes and moved footrests out of the way.	___	___
7. Lowered bed, locked wheels, and lowered rail on side of bed.*	___	___
8. Assisted client, as needed, to sit on side of bed and put on robe and footwear.	___	___
9. Stood directly in front of client, with feet slightly apart. Bent hips and knees to be level with client.	___	___
10. Placed arms under client's arms and around client's back, locking fingers together or clasping one hand over the other wrist. Asked client to hug aide's back or shoulders.	___	___
11. Locked knees against client's to provide additional support and to prevent the knees from buckling.	___	___
12. Bent knees and asked client to rock with aide while counting 1-2-3. Stood on the count of "3."	___	___
13. Counted to 10 before continuing to allow the client time to adjust to standing position.	___	___
14. Walked with client to chair (took small steps) and guided client's back to chair. Continued until chair's sitting surface touched back of client's legs.	___	___
15. Had client reach back and grasp the farthest arm of the chair, then the nearest arm.	___	___
16. Bent hips and knees while guiding client into chair.	___	___
17. Made sure client was safe and comfortable.	___	___
a. If in wheelchair, replaced footrests and had client put feet on them.	___	___
b. Placed necessary items within client's reach.	___	___
18. Washed hands.	___	___
19. Recorded client's reaction to procedure, amount of time spent sitting in chair, and any other observations	___	___

Comments:

Evaluator's Signature: _____
Date: _____

*Will not apply if hospital bed is not used.

Procedure 12-12.   Transferring Client From Bed to Chair/Wheelchair—Standing Transfer Using Transfer Belt

Name: _____

	S	UN
1. Explained procedure to client.	___	___
2. Washed hands.	___	___
3. Obtained materials needed.	___	___
4. Provided privacy.	___	___
5. Applied transfer belt.	___	___
6. Placed chair parallel to bed and on client's strong side. If wheelchair was used, locked brakes and moved footrests out of the way. If bed has wheels, locked them.	___	___
7. Stood directly in front of client.	___	___
8. Made sure client's feet were firmly on the floor.	___	___
9. Had client place fists on bed next to thighs and lean forward.	___	___
10. Grasped transfer belt firmly at each side.	___	___
11. Locked knees against client's knees to provide additional support and to prevent client's knees from buckling.	___	___
12. Asked client to push fists down on bed and stand on count of "3".	___	___
13. Pulled client to standing position while straightening knees and legs.	___	___
14. Counted to 10 before continuing.	___	___
15. Instructed client to:	___	___
a. Take small steps while turning back to chair until legs touch the chair.	___	___
b. Reach back and grasp the farthest arm of the chair, then the nearest arm.	___	___
c. Lower buttocks into chair, leaning slightly forward while sitting down.	___	___
d. Slide hips and back into chair and sit erect.	___	___
16. Made sure client was safe and comfortable.	___	___
a. If in wheelchair, replaced footrests and had client put feet on them.	___	___
b. Placed necessary items within client's reach.	___	___
17. Washed hands.	___	___
18. Recorded client's reaction to procedure, amount of time spent sitting in chair, and any other observations	___	___

Comments:

Evaluator's Signature: _____
Date: _____

*Will not apply if hospital bed is not used.

Procedure 12-13.   Returning Client to Bed

Name: _____

	S	UN
1. Explained procedure to client.	____	____
2. Washed hands.	____	____
3. Provided privacy.	____	____
4. Prepared the bed; folded down top bedding.	____	____
5. Lowered height of bed to lowest level*	____	____
6. Placed chair parallel to bed—client moved toward strong side.	____	____
7. Locked brakes and moved foot rests out of way, if wheelchair is used. Locked bed wheels (if present).	____	____
8. Directed client to:	____	____
a. Hold on to armrests.	____	____
b. Slide to edge of chair.	____	____
c. Push down on armrests, straighten legs, and stand up.	____	____
d. Take small steps while turning back to bed until back of legs touch the bed.	____	____
e. Reach back and place hands on bed.	____	____
f. Lower buttocks onto bed and slide back in bed.	____	____
9. Assisted client to remove robe and shoes.	____	____
10. Made sure client was safe and comfortable.	____	____
11. Placed bed in lowest position. (Raised side rails, if indicated.)*	____	____
12. Washed hands.	____	____
13. Recorded what was done and client's reaction.	____	____

Comments:

Evaluator's Signature: _____

Date: _____

*Will not apply if hospital bed is not used.

Procedure 12-14.　　Applying a Transfer (Gait) Belt

Name: _____

	S	UN
1. Explained procedure to client.	____	____
2. Washed hands.	____	____
3. Obtained transfer (gait) belt	____	____
4. Assisted client to sitting position on side of bed.	____	____
5. Applied belt over clothing and around waist.	____	____
6. Placed belt buckles off-center in the front or in the back according to client's comfort.	____	____
7. Tightened belt, using buckles, until it is snug.	____	____
8. Check that breasts (women) are not caught in the belt.	____	____
9. Prepared client for transfer.	____	____

Comments:

Evaluator's Signature: _____
Date: _____

Procedure 12-15.   Using a Mechanical Lift

Name: _____

	S	UN
1. Explained procedure to client.	___	___
2. Washed hands.	___	___
3. Obtained necessary materials.	___	___
4. Provided privacy.	___	___
5. Raised bed to convenient working height and lowered side rails.*	___	___
6. Lowered head of bed to level comfortable for client—as low as possible.*	___	___
7. Centered sling with sheet on top, placing them underneath client by turning client from side to side.	___	___
8. Positioned sling according to manufacturer's instructions.	___	___
9. Placed chair/wheelchair at head or foot of bed, about 1 foot away from side of bed.	___	___
10. Locked wheels on bed.*	___	___
11. Raised lift and positioned over client.	___	___
12. Rolled base of lift under bed, locating swivel bar over client.	___	___
13. Attached sling to swivel bar.	___	___
14. Raised head of bed to sitting position.*	___	___
15. Placed client's arms across chest. Client did not touch swivel bar.	___	___
16. Pumped lift high enough for client and sling to be free of the bed.	___	___
17. Asked helper to support client's legs and guide client as lift was moved and client moved away from bed.	___	___
18. Positioned lift so that client's back was toward chair.	___	___
19. Lowered client into chair as helper guided client into chair. Followed manufacturer's instructions for lowering lift.	___	___
20. Lowered the swivel bar to unhook the sling. Left the sling in place.	___	___
21. Put on client's footwear; positioned feet.	___	___
22. Covered client's lap and legs with blanket, as needed.	___	___
23. Made sure client was safe and comfortable.	___	___
24. Washed hands.	___	___
25. Recorded client's reaction to procedure, amount of time spent sitting in chair, and any other observations.	___	___
26. Reversed procedure to return client to bed.	___	___

Comments:

Evaluator's Signature: _____
Date: _____

*Will not apply if hospital bed is not used.

Procedure 13-1. Making a Closed Bed

Name: _____

	S	UN
1. Explained procedure to client.	___	___
2. Washed hands.	___	___
3. Obtained materials needed and placed them in order of use on chair near bed.	___	___
4. Placed laundry container near bed.	___	___
5. Raised bed to convenient working height and lowered both rails.*	___	___
6. Placed bed in flat position.*	___	___
7. Removed pillow(s) and placed on chair.	___	___
8. Loosened all bed linens — at head, sides, and bottom of bed.	___	___
9. Removed each piece of bed linen separately. Folded any linens to be reused. Rolled each remaining linen into a ball and discarded in laundry container.	___	___
10. Placed clean mattress pad, folded lengthwise, in center of bed. Unfolded one half and rolled to center of bed[†]	___	___
11. Placed bottom sheet, folded lengthwise, in center of bed. Unfolded one half and rolled to center of bed.	___	___
a. Fitted sheet — placed ends around corners — top and bottom; tucked side of sheet under mattress	___	___
b. Flat sheet — placed bottom hem of sheet even with edge of mattress at foot of bed; tucked top of sheet under mattress at head of bed.	___	___
12. Mitered corner at head of mattress.	___	___
13. Tucked sheet under side of entire mattress. Worked from head of bed to foot.	___	___
14. Placed plastic drawsheet, folded in half, in center third of bed.[†]	___	___
15. Placed cotton drawsheet, folded in half, in center of bed, covering entire plastic drawsheet. Unfolded and rolled to center of bed.[†]	___	___
16. Tucked ends of plastic drawsheet and cotton drawsheet under mattress.[†]	___	___
17. Placed top sheet, folded lengthwise, in center of bed, with top edge even with top of mattress. Unfolded and rolled to center of bed.	___	___
18. Placed blanket, folded lengthwise, in center of bed, with top edge even with top of mattress. Unfolded and rolled to center of bed.[†]	___	___
19. Placed bedspread, folded lengthwise, in center of bed, with about 4 inches above top edge of mattress. Unfolded and rolled to center of bed.[†]	___	___
20. Tucked top sheet, blanket, and bedspread under foot of mattress. Mitered corner.	___	___
21. Went to other side of bed	___	___

	S	UN
22. Pulled through mattress pad and straightened.[†]	___	___
23. Pulled through all lower linens. Straightened and tucked under mattress. Mitered corner of sheet at head of bed. (Or placed top and bottom corners of fitted sheet over mattress corners.)	___	___
24. Pulled through top sheet, blanket, and spread. Smoothed out wrinkles.	___	___
25. Tucked top sheet, blanket, and bedspread under foot of mattress.	___	___
26. Mitered corner at foot of bed.	___	___
27. Made a cuff at top of bed and brought top sheet over blanket.	___	___
28. Placed clean pillowcase on pillow and placed pillow at head of bed.	___	___
29. Covered pillow with bedspread.	___	___
30. Placed bed in lowest position.*	___	___
31. Removed laundry container and took to washing machine or other location as requested by client or family.	___	___
32. Washed hands.	___	___

Comments:

Evaluator's Signature: _____
Date: _____

*Will not apply if hospital bed is not used.
[†]Optional.

Procedure 13-2.   Making an Open Bed

Name: _____

	S	UN
1. Washed hands.	____	____
2. Obtained necessary materials.	____	____
3. Made a closed bed.	____	____
4. Fanfolded top linens to foot of bed.	____	____
5. Washed hands.	____	____

Comments:

Evaluator's Signature: _____
Date: _____

Procedure 13-3.   Making an Occupied Bed

Name: _____

	S	UN
1. Explained procedure to client.	___	___
2. Washed hands.	___	___
3. Obtained materials needed and placed them in order of use on chair near bed.	___	___
4. Provided privacy.	___	___
5. Placed laundry container near bed.	___	___
6. Raised bed to convenient working height and locked wheels. Lowered rail on side of bed where aide is to work.*	___	___
7. Lowered head of bed to level comfortable for client—as low as possible*	___	___
8. Loosened top bedding at foot of bed.	___	___
9. Removed top bedding (bedspread, quilt), but left client covered with one blanket or top sheet.	___	___
10. Instructed client to hold top sheet while other top linens are removed.	___	___
11. Folded any linens to be reused, such as blanket or quilt. Rolled each remaining linen into a ball and discarded in laundry container.	___	___
12. Helped client to roll to side of bed opposite aide and grasp side rail for support.*	___	___
13. Rolled each piece of bottom linen to center of bed and tucked along client's back.	___	___
14. Smoothed mattress pad, if used.†	___	___
15. Placed clean bottom sheet, folded lengthwise, in center of bed. Unfolded one half and rolled to center of bed.	___	___
a. Fitted sheet—placed ends around corners—top and bottom; tucked side of sheet under mattress.	___	___
b. Flat sheet—placed bottom hem of sheet even with edge of mattress at foot of bed; tucked top of sheet under mattress at head of bed.	___	___
16. Mitered corner at head of mattress.	___	___
17. Tucked sheet under side of entire mattress. Worked from head of bed to foot.	___	___
18. Placed plastic drawsheet, folded in half, in center third of bed. Unfolded and rolled to center of bed. Tucked along client's back.†	___	___
19. Placed cotton drawsheet, folded in half, in center of bed, covering entire plastic drawsheet. Unfolded and rolled to center of bed. Tucked along client's back.	___	___
20. Tucked ends of drawsheet(s) under mattress.†	___	___
21. Helped client to roll toward aide, over linens to clean side of bed.	___	___
22. Raised rail on side where aide will work.*	___	___
23. Went to other side of bed.	___	___
24. Lowered side rail.*	___	___

	S	**UN**
25. Removed used bottom linens, rolled and discarded in laundry container.	___	___
26. Pulled through all bottom linens. Straightened and tucked under head of mattress. Mitered corner of sheet at head of bed. (Or fitted top and bottom corners of fitted sheet over mattress corners.)	___	___
27. Helped client to roll back to center of bed.	___	___
28. Placed clean top sheet entirely over the client and removed top linens; discarded in laundry container or folded for reuse.	___	___
29. Placed blanket and bedspread over sheet.	___	___
30. Tucked top sheet, blanket, and bedspread under foot of mattress. Made a mitered corner.	___	___
31. Raised side rail.*	___	___
32. Went to other side of bed. Lowered side rail.*	___	___
33. Smoothed and straightened top sheet, blanket, and bedspread. Tucked them under foot of mattress. Made mitered corner.	___	___
34. Made cuff at top of bed and brought top sheet over bedspread.	___	___
35. Removed pillow from bed, took off case and discarded in laundry container.	___	___
36. Applied clean pillowcase; placed pillow under client's head.	___	___
37. Made sure client was safe and comfortable.	___	___
38. Placed bed in lowest position. (Raise side rail if indicated.)*	___	___
39. Removed laundry container to proper location.	___	___
40. Washed hands.	___	___

Comments:

Evaluator's Signature: _____
Date: _____

*Will not apply if hospital bed is not used.
†Optional.

Procedure 13-4.   Making a Mitered Corner

Name: _____

BOTTOM BEDDING

	S	UN
1. Tucked bottom sheet about 18 inches under the mattress at head of bed.	___	___
2. Turned side of sheet up over the mattress in a triangle shape.	___	___
3. Tucked the lower edge of the sheet (hanging down next to the mattress) under the side of the mattress.	___	___
4. Turned the triangular area of sheet down over the mattress.	___	___
5. Tucked sheet under the mattress.	___	___

Comments:

Evaluator's Signature: _____
Date: _____

Procedure 14-1.   Brushing Teeth

Name: _____

	S	UN
1. Explained procedure to client.	____	____
2. Washed hands.	____	____
3. Obtained necessary materials.	____	____
4. Provided privacy.	____	____
5. Spread paper towel on work area. Arranged supplies on paper towel.	____	____
6. Raised bed to convenient working height. Lowered rail on side of bed.*	____	____
7. Assisted client to an upright position, or turned on side if unable to sit up.	____	____
8. Placed face towel under client's chin and over chest.	____	____
9. Put on gloves.	____	____
10. Assisted client with self-care as necessary.	____	____
11. Held toothbrush over emesis basis and poured a little water over the brush to moisten. Applied toothpaste.	____	____
12. Brushed client's teeth (if client is unable to do so).	____	____
13. Had client rinse mouth with water. Held emesis basin so client could spit into it.	____	____
14. Had client rinse with mouthwash (optional). Held emesis basin so client could spit into it.	____	____
15. Wiped client's mouth with face towel.	____	____
16. Removed face towel.	____	____
17. Removed and discarded gloves.	____	____
18. Made sure client was safe and comfortable.	____	____
19. Placed bed in lowest position. (Raised side rail, if indicated.)*	____	____
20. Cleaned equipment and stored in proper location.	____	____
21. Wiped work surface with paper towel and discarded.	____	____
22. Placed soiled face towel in laundry container to be washed.	____	____
23. Washed hands.	____	____
24. Recorded what was done. Reported any unusual conditions to supervisor.	____	____

Comments:

Evaluator's Signature: _____
Date: _____

*Will not apply if hospital bed is not used.

Procedure 14-2.   Flossing Teeth

Name: _____

	S	UN
1. Explained procedure to client.	___	___
2. Washed hands.	___	___
3. Obtained necessary materials.	___	___
4. Provided privacy.	___	___
5. Spread paper towel on work area. Arranged supplies on paper towel.	___	___
6. Raised bed to convenient working height. Lowered rail on side.*	___	___
7. Assisted client to an upright position, or turned on side if unable to sit up.	___	___
8. Placed face towel under client's chin and over chest.	___	___
9. Put on gloves.	___	___
10. Removed 18 inches (44-46 cm) of floss from dispenser.	___	___
11. Wrapped floss around the middle finger of each hand to clean upper teeth.	___	___
12. Held floss with index fingers to clean lower teeth.	___	___
13. Inserted floss between teeth and used up and down, back and forth motions to remove material between teeth. Proceeded from tooth to tooth:	___	___
a. Upper teeth, left to right	___	___
b. Lower teeth, left to right	___	___
14. Had client rinse mouth with water. Held emesis basin so client could spit into it.	___	___
15. Wiped client's mouth with face towel.	___	___
16. Removed face towel.	___	___
17. Removed and discarded gloves.	___	___
18. Made sure client was safe and comfortable.	___	___
19. Placed bed in lowest position. (Raised side rail, if indicated.)*	___	___
20. Cleaned equipment and stored in proper location.	___	___
21. Wiped work surface with paper towel and discarded.	___	___
22. Placed soiled face towel in laundry container to be washed.	___	___
23. Washed hands.	___	___
24. Recorded what was done. Reported any unusual conditions to supervisor.	___	___

Comments:

Evaluator's Signature: _____
Date: _____

*Will not apply if hospital bed is not used.

Procedure 14-3. Mouth Care for the Unconscious Client

Name: _____

	S	UN
1. Explained procedure to client.	___	___
2. Washed hands.	___	___
3. Obtained necessary materials.	___	___
4. Provided privacy.	___	___
5. Spread paper towel on work area. Arranged supplies on paper towel.	___	___
6. Raised bed to convenient working height. Lowered rail on side.*	___	___
7. Placed client in a side-lying position.	___	___
8. Placed face towel and emesis basin under client's chin.	___	___
9. Put on gloves.	___	___
10. Gently opened client's mouth with padded tongue depressor.	___	___
11. Moistened foam swab and cleaned all surfaces of mouth: roof of mouth, tongue, gums, lips, inside of cheeks. Rinsed and re-wet swab as necessary. Cleaned teeth with swab.	___	___
12. Wiped client's mouth with face towel.	___	___
13. Removed face towel.	___	___
14. Applied lubricant to lips.	___	___
15. Removed and discarded gloves.	___	___
16. Made sure client was safe and comfortable.	___	___
17. Placed bed in lowest position. (Raised side rail, if indicated.)*	___	___
18. Cleaned equipment and stored in proper location.	___	___
19. Wiped work surface with paper towel and discarded.	___	___
20. Placed soiled face towel in laundry container to be washed.	___	___
21. Washed hands.	___	___
22. Recorded what was done. Reported any unusual conditions to supervisor.	___	___

Comments:

Evaluator's Signature: _____
Date: _____

*Will not apply if hospital bed is not used.

Procedure 14-4.   Caring for Dentures

Name: _____

	S	UN
1. Explained procedure to client.		
2. Washed hands.	___	___
3. Obtained necessary materials.	___	___
4. Provided privacy.	___	___
5. Spread paper towel on work area. Arranged supplies on paper towel (if procedure performed at bedside). Otherwise, took supplies for cleaning dentures to sink.	___	___
6. Raised bed to convenient working height. Lowered rail on side.*	___	___
7. Assisted client to an upright position or turned on side, if unable to sit up.	___	___
8. Put on gloves.	___	___
9. Asked client to remove dentures and placed in emesis basin. If dentures must be removed, used gauze or a tissue as follows:	___	___
a. Upper dentures: Grasped between thumb and index finger and moved up and down gently. Pulled down and removed.	___	___
b. Lower dentures: Grasped in the same manner and gently twisted sideways and up, lifting them out of the mouth.	___	___
10. Assisted client to brush dentures.	___	___
11. Cleaned dentures at sink:		
a. Partially filled sink with warm water.	___	___
b. Brushed with warm water and toothpaste in an up-and-down motion. Rinsed thoroughly.	___	___
12. Returned dentures to client for replacement in the mouth or stored in denture cup.	___	___
13. Removed and discarded gloves.	___	___
14. Made sure client was safe and comfortable.	___	___
15. Placed bed in lowest position. (Raised side rail, if indicated.)*	___	___
16. Cleaned equipment and stored in proper location.	___	___
17. Wiped work surface with paper towel and discarded.	___	___
18. Washed hands.	___	___
19. Recorded what was done. Reported any unusual conditions to supervisor.	___	___

Comments:

Evaluator's Signature: _____
Date: _____

*Will not apply if hospital bed is not used.

Procedure 14-5.   Giving a Complete Bed Bath

Name: _____

	S	UN
1. Explained procedure to client.	____	____
2. Washed hands.	____	____
3. Obtained necessary materials.	____	____
4. Provided privacy.	____	____
5. Raised bed to convenient working height. Locked wheels. Lowered rail on side.*	____	____
6. Offered bed pan or urinal.	____	____
7. Lowered head of bed to level comfortable for client—as low as possible.*	____	____
8. Removed top bedding and covered client with bath blanket or top sheet.	____	____
9. Helped client to remove clothing, if needed.	____	____
10. Helped client to move to side of bed near aide.	____	____
11. Helped client with oral hygiene, if needed.	____	____
12. Filled wash basin two-thirds full with warm water (110°-115° F; 43°-46° C).	____	____
13. Placed towel under client's head and towel over client's chest.	____	____
14. Made a mitt with washcloth to be used throughout procedure.	____	____
15. Washed eye areas gently with clean water only. Started from inner corner of eye to outer corner of eye. Used opposite corners of washcloth for each eye.	____	____
16. Asked client if he or she preferred soap or cleansing cream to clean face.	____	____
17. Washed face from center outward. Used firm, gentle movements.	____	____
18. Washed ears and neck. Rinsed and dried using towel on client's chest.	____	____
19. Put a towel, lengthwise, under the arm and a towel near hand on which to place the wash basin.	____	____
20. Put client's hand in basin; allowed it to soak. Washed the arm and armpit.	____	____
21. Washed, rinsed, and dried arm, armpit, and hand. Applied deodorant under the arm, if requested. Pushed back cuticles; cleaned under nails with orangewood stick. Dried between fingers thoroughly.	____	____
22. Followed steps 19 to 21 for the other arm and hand.	____	____
23. Placed basin back on bedside table or chair.	____	____
24. Put towel over chest and abdomen. Pulled bath blanket (top sheet) to thighs. Did not expose client when washing chest and abdomen.	____	____
25. Washed, rinsed, and dried chest and abdomen. Covered chest and abdomen with bath blanket (top sheet). Removed towel.	____	____
26. Uncovered leg. Did not expose genital area. Placed towel under the leg and foot. Placed another towel near foot and put basin on towel.	____	____
27. Bent client's knee and put foot in basin; allowed it to soak. Washed and dried leg while foot was soaking.	____	____

	S	UN
28. Washed and dried foot. Cleaned under toenails. Dried between toes thoroughly.	___	___
29. Repeated steps 26 to 28 for other leg and foot.	___	___
30. Placed basin back on bedside table or chair.	___	___
31. Turned client on side; draped bath blanket (top sheet) and exposed back and buttocks.	___	___
32. Placed towel on bed, tucked lengthwise along neck and shoulders to buttocks.	___	___
33. Washed, rinsed, and dried neck, shoulders, back, and buttocks. Worked from neck to buttocks. Used long strokes for washing the back.	___	___
34. Gave back rub.	___	___
35. Changed bath water.	___	___
36. Turned client onto back.	___	___
37. Placed towel under buttocks. Placed basin, soap, and towels within reach. Had client wash genital and rectal areas. Asked client to tell you when this was complete. If client was unable to wash these areas, aide completed this part of the bath wearing disposable gloves.	___	___
38. Helped client to put on gown, pajamas, or other clothing.	___	___
39. Combed or brushed client's hair.	___	___
40. Made sure client was safe and comfortable.	___	___
41. Placed bed in lowest position. (Raised side rail, if indicated.)*	___	___
42. Emptied and cleaned wash basin. Wiped off work area with paper towels and discarded. Placed soiled towels and washcloth in laundry container to be washed. Returned other supplies to their proper place.	___	___
43. Washed hands.	___	___
44. Recorded what was done. Reported any unusual conditions to supervisor.	___	___

Comments:

Evaluator's Signature: _____
Date: _____

*Will not apply if hospital bed is not used.

Procedure 14-6.   Giving a Tub Bath

Name: _____

		S	UN
1.	Explained procedure to client.	___	___
2.	Washed hands.	___	___
3.	Obtained necessary materials.	___	___
4.	Prepared bathroom by placing skid-proof mat on bottom of tub, making sure room was warm and free of drafts, and placing straight chair in bathroom.	___	___
5.	Provided privacy.	___	___
6.	Helped client to undress; put on bathrobe and footwear. Placed client in wheelchair, if used. Locked brakes and put footrests in place.	___	___
7.	Filled tub one-third full of warm water (110°-115° F; 43°-46° C).	___	___
8.	Helped client to bathroom and closed door.	___	___
9.	Placed client in chair facing tub. If wheelchair was used, locked brakes and placed footrests out of the way.	___	___
10.	Helped client to lift one foot, then the other, over the side of the tub.	___	___
11.	Helped client to lower into water, used grab bars for support.	___	___
12.	Helped client to bathe as needed.	___	___
13.	Drained water from tub before getting client out of tub.	___	___
14.	Helped client to dry body. Assisted client to put on bathrobe or covered with dry towel.	___	___
15.	Placed straight chair or wheelchair facing tub and placed dry towel on side of tub.	___	___
16.	Helped client to sit on towel on side of tub using grab bars.	___	___
17.	Helped client to stand, get out of tub into straight chair or wheelchair, and put on footwear.	___	___
18.	Helped client to room.	___	___
19.	Gave back rub.	___	___
20.	Helped client to put on clean clothing and returned to bed, sofa, etc. Placed in comfortable position.	___	___
21.	Made sure client was safe and comfortable.	___	___
22.	Returned to bathroom. Cleaned tub and straightened area.	___	___
23.	Placed soiled towels and washcloth in laundry container to be washed.	___	___
24.	Washed hands.		___
25.	Recorded what was done. Reported any unusual conditions to supervisor.	___	___

Comments:

Evaluator's Signature: _____
Date: _____

Procedure 14-7.   Giving a Back Rub

Name: _____

	S	UN
1. Explained procedure to client.	___	___
2. Washed hands.	___	___
3. Obtained necessary materials.	___	___
4. Provided privacy.	___	___
5. Raised bed to convenient working height and locked wheels. Lowered rail on side.*	___	___
6. Lowered head of bed to a level comfortable for client—as low as possible.*	___	___
7. Removed clothing from upper body.	___	___
8. Placed client on side or abdomen to expose entire back.	___	___
9. Put small amount of lotion on hands. Rubbed hands together to warm lotion.	___	___
10. Used correct body mechanics. Faced head of bed, one foot slightly forward, knees bent.	___	___
11. Started at the lower back and moved upward toward the shoulders. Applied pressure using palms of both hands. Used long, firm but gentle strokes: up, out, and down. Repeated several times.	___	___
12. Removed excess lotion with towel.	___	___
13. Helped client to put on clothes.	___	___
14. Made sure client was safe and comfortable.	___	___
15. Placed bed in lowest position. (Raised side rail, if indicated.)*	___	___
16. Washed hands.	___	___
17. Recorded what was done. Reported any unusual conditions to supervisor.	___	___

Comments:

Evaluator's Signature: _____
Date: _____

*Will not apply if hospital bed is not used.

Procedure 14-8.   Giving Perineal Care

Name: _____

	S	UN
1. Explained procedure to client.	___	___
2. Washed hands.	___	___
3. Obtained necessary materials.	___	___
4. Spread paper towel on work area. Arranged supplies on paper towel.	___	___
5. Provided privacy.	___	___
6. Raised bed to convenient working height. Lowered rail on side.*	___	___
7. Folded top bedding to foot of bed and covered client with sheet or blanket.	___	___
8. Helped client into supine position and removed clothing from waist down.	___	___
9. Positioned waterproof protector pad(s) under buttocks.	___	___
10. Draped the client.	___	___
11. Raised side rail.*	___	___
12. Filled wash basin two-thirds full with warm water (105°-110° F; 41°-43° C).	___	___
13. Placed basin on work area on top of paper towels.	___	___
14. Lowered rail on side where work will be done.*	___	___
15. Folded back the corner of blanket or sheet between client's legs and onto abdomen.	___	___
16. Helped client to bend knees and spread legs.	___	___
17. Put on disposable gloves.	___	___
18. Applied soap and water to washcloth or cotton balls.	___	___
19. Provided female perineal care:	___	___
a. Separated labia.	___	___
b. Cleaned downward, with one stroke, from front to back. Used clean washcloth or cotton ball for each stroke. Put used cotton balls in bag or set aside used washcloths. Repeated this step until area was clean.	___	___
c. Rinsed area, using same procedure as in steps 19a and 19b.	___	___
d. Dried area thoroughly.	___	___
e. Folded blanket back between client's legs.	___	___
f. Helped client to straighten legs and turn on side away from aide.	___	___
g. Separated buttocks and cleaned rectal area with toilet tissue, if needed. Washed area from vagina to anus, using clean washcloth for each stroke. Repeated this step until area was clean.	___	___
h. Rinsed area, using same procedure as in step 19g.	___	___
i. Dried area.	___	___
20. Provided male perineal care:		
a. Gently pulled back foreskin, if client is uncircumcised.	___	___
b. While holding penis, cleaned tip, using circular motion. Started at the urethral opening and worked outward. Repeated this step, using a clean washcloth or cotton ball, until area was clean. Put used cotton balls in bag or set aside used washcloths.	___	___

	S	UN

c. Rinsed and dried area thoroughly, using same procedure as steps 20*a* and 20*b*. ____ ____

d. Returned foreskin to natural position if client is uncircumcised. ____ ____

e. Cleaned shaft of penis using washcloth with firm but gentle downward strokes. Rinsed and dried area thoroughly. ____ ____

f. Helped client to bend knees and spread legs. ____ ____

g. Gently cleaned scrotum. Washed skin folds carefully. Rinsed and dried area thoroughly. ____ ____

h. Helped client to straighten legs and turn on side away from aide. ____ ____

i. Separated buttocks and cleaned rectal area with toilet tissue, if needed. ____ ____

Washed from scrotum to anus using clean washcloth for each stroke. Repeated this step until area was clean. ____ ____

j. Rinsed area using same procedure as in step 20*i*. ____ ____

k. Dried area. ____ ____

21. Removed soiled bedding, washcloths, and waterproof protector pad and placed in laundry container. ____ ____

22. Removed gloves and discarded into bag. ____ ____

23. Straightened bedding; removed sheet or blanket. ____ ____

24. Made sure client was safe and comfortable. ____ ____

25. Placed bed in lowest position. (Raised side rail, if indicated.)* ____ ____

26. Emptied and cleaned washbasin. Wiped off work area with paper towels and discarded into bag. Returned other materials to their proper place. ____ ____

27. Washed hands. ____ ____

28. Recorded what was done. Reported any unusual conditions to supervisor. ____ ____

Comments:

Evaluator's Signature: _____
Date: _____

*Will not apply if hospital bed is not used.

Procedure 14-9.   Caring for Nails and Feet

Name: _____

	S	UN
1. Explained procedure to client.	___	___
2. Washed hands.	___	___
3. Obtained necessary materials.	___	___
4. Spread paper towel on work area. Arranged supplies on paper towel.	___	___
5. Provided privacy.	___	___
6. Helped client into chair or to side of bed.	___	___
7. Assisted client to remove footwear, if appropriate.	___	___
8. Put bath mat, towel, or newspapers under feet.	___	___
9. Filled basin with warm water (100°-110° F; 38°-43° C).	___	___
10. Placed basin on bath mat. Put on gloves (optional). Helped client put feet in basin.	___	___
11. Allowed feet to soak for 10 minutes. Added warm water as needed.	___	___
12. Placed table or ironing board in front of client at convenient height and close to client. Covered table with hand towel or paper towels.	___	___
13. Filled emesis basin or small bowl with water (100°-110° F; 38°-43° C) Put client's fingers in basin and soaked for 2 to 3 minutes.	___	___
14. Cleaned under fingernails with orangewood stick. Dried fingers thoroughly and set basin aside.	___	___
15. Shaped fingernails with emery board or nail file. Pushed back cuticles gently with washcloth or orangewood stick. Applied hand lotion (optional).	___	___
16. Removed table.	___	___
17. Removed one foot from basin. Smoothed any calloused areas using washcloth or pumice stone. Dried foot and between toes thoroughly. Repeated procedure for other foot. Applied lotion, as needed.	___	___
18. Removed gloves, if worn, and discarded.	___	___
19. Helped client to put on footwear or helped back to bed.	___	___
20. Cleaned equipment and stored in proper location. Discarded disposable supplies.	___	___
21. Placed soiled towels in laundry container to be washed.	___	___
22. Washed hands.	___	___
23. Recorded what was done. Reported any unusual conditions to supervisor.		___

Comments:

Evaluator's Signature: _____
Date: _____

Procedure 14-10.   Assisting Client With Hair Care

Name: _____

	S	UN
1. Explained procedure to client.	___	___
2. Washed hands.	___	___
3. Obtained necessary materials.	___	___
4. Provided privacy.	___	___
5. Raised bed to convenient working height. Lowered rail on side of bed where aide is working.*	___	___
6. Placed client in upright position in bed or in chair, if possible.	___	___
7. Placed bath towel around client's shoulders. If the client is in bed, placed towel under head to cover the pillow.	___	___
8. Parted hair and separated into sections.	___	___
9. Brushed hair, section by section; worked from root to end of hair.	___	___
10. Arranged hair according to client's wishes.	___	___
11. Removed towel.	___	___
12. Made sure client was safe and comfortable.	___	___
13. Placed bed in lowest position.*	___	___
14. Cleaned supplies and stored in proper location.	___	___
15. Placed soiled bath towel in laundry container to be washed.	___	___
16. Washed hands.	___	___
17. Recorded what was done. Reported any unusual conditions to supervisor.	___	___

Comments:

Evaluator's Signature: _____
Date: _____

*Will not apply if hospital bed is not used.

Procedure 14-11.   Giving a Shampoo

Name: _____

	S	UN
1. Explained procedure to client.	____	____
2. Washed hands.	____	____
3. Obtained necessary materials.	____	____
4. Provided privacy. Removed glasses, hearing aids. Stored properly.	____	____
5. Raised bed to convenient working height. Lowered rail on side of bed where aide is working.*	____	____
6. Positioned client for shampoo—at sink, in tub or shower, or in bed with trough under head and neck.	____	____
7. Brushed and combed hair.	____	____
8. Had client hold folded washcloth over eyes to protect from shampoo.	____	____
9. Wet hair, from front to back, with warm water (100° F; 38° C).	____	____
10. Put a small amount of shampoo in palm of hand.	____	____
11. Applied shampoo to scalp; lathered from front to back, rubbed gently.	____	____
12. Rinsed thoroughly with warm water.	____	____
13. Repeated steps 10 through 12.	____	____
14. Applied conditioner, according to direction, as desired.	____	____
15. Wrapped client's head in bath towel.	____	____
16. Bath/shower stall—Helped client out and assisted with drying body and hair.	____	____
17. Bed shampoo—Removed trough from bed. Towel dried hair.	____	____
18. Dried hair using hair dryer, if available. Arranged hair according to client's wishes.	____	____
19. Made sure client was safe and comfortable. Replaced eye glasses, hearing aids, if appropriate.	____	____
20. Placed bed in lowest position. (Raised side rail, if indicated.)*	____	____
21. Cleaned materials and stored in proper location.	____	____
22. Placed soiled bath towel in laundry container.	____	____
23. Washed hands.	____	____
24. Recorded what was done. Reported any unusual conditions to supervisor.	____	____

Comments:

Evaluator's Signature: _____
Date: _____

*Will not apply if hospital bed is not used.

Procedure 14-12.   Shaving the Male Client

Name: _____

	S	UN
1. Explained procedure to client.	____	____
2. Washed hands.	____	____
3. Obtained necessary materials.	____	____
4. Provided privacy.	____	____
5. Raised bed to convenient working height. Lowered rail on side of bed.*	____	____
6. Placed client in an upright position in bed (or assisted to sit by bathroom sink, if possible).	____	____
7. Shaving with a blade razor:	____	____
a. Put on disposable gloves.	____	____
b. Wet washcloth with warm water (115° F; 46° C). Placed on client's face for a few minutes. Removed.	____	____
c. Applied shaving cream and lathered the face.	____	____
d. Held the skin taut and shaved in the direction of hair growth.	____	____
e. Rinsed razor blade when necessary.	____	____
f. Rinsed skin and dried with towel.	____	____
8. Shaving with an electric razor:	____	____
a. Put on disposable gloves.	____	____
b. Made sure face was clean and dry.	____	____
c. Turned on razor.	____	____
d. Held skin taut and shaved in the direction of hair growth.	____	____
e. Turned off razor.	____	____
9. Removed towel.	____	____
10. Removed and discarded gloves.	____	____
11. Made sure client was safe and comfortable.	____	____
12. Placed bed in lowest position. (Raised side rail if indicated.)*	____	____
13. Cleaned materials and stored in proper location.	____	____
14. Placed soiled linens in laundry container.	____	____
15. Washed hands.	____	____
16. Recorded what was done. Reported any unusual conditions to supervisor.	____	____

Comments:

Evaluator's Signature: _____
Date: _____

*Will not apply if hospital bed is not used.

Procedure 14-13. Helping Client to Dress

Name: _____

	S	UN
1. Explained procedure to client.	___	___
2. Washed hands.	___	___
3. Obtained necessary materials.	___	___
4. Arranged clothing in order of use.	___	___
5. Provided privacy.	___	___
6. Lowered bed to lowest position. Lowered rail on side of bed.*	___	___
7. Helped client to sit on side of bed, if possible. If client must stay in bed, placed in supine position.	___	___
8. Helped client to put on undershirt or bra, shirt, or pajama top.	___	___
a. Over-the-head type garment—Placed injured arm into garment first. Pulled neck of garment over client's head. Guided other arm into garment.	___	___
b. Front-button or zipping type garment—Placed injured arm through sleeve first. Brought shirt to the back of client and guided the other arm into the sleeve.	___	___
9. Helped client to put on underwear, slacks, shorts, or pajama bottoms. If leg is injured, placed into garment first, then the other leg. Helped client to stand at side of bed and pulled up clothing to the waist. If client is in bed, helped client to lift buttocks and (aide) pulled up garments.	___	___
10. Helped client to put on socks or stockings and footwear.	___	___
11. Made sure client was safe and comfortable.	___	___
12. Placed bed in lowest position. (Raised side rail, if indicated).*	___	___
13. Washed hands.	___	___
14. Recorded what was done. Reported any unusual conditions to supervisor.	___	___

Comments:

Evaluator's Signature: _____
Date: _____

*Will not apply if hospital bed is not used.

Procedure 14-14.   Helping Client With an IV to Remove Used Clothing and Apply Clean Clothing

Name: _____

	S	UN
1. Explained procedure to client.	____	____
2. Washed hands.	____	____
3. Obtained necessary materials.	____	____
4. Arranged clothing in order of use.	____	____
5. Provided privacy.	____	____
6. Lowered bed to lowest position. Lowered rail on side of bed.*	____	____
7. Helped client to sit on side of bed, if possible. If client must stay in bed, placed in supine position.	____	____
8. Helped client to remove used garment from arm without IV.	____	____
9. Gathered up sleeve of garment on arm with IV. Slid sleeve over the IV site and tubing. Removed client's arm and hand from the sleeve.	____	____
10. Slid hand along tubing to IV bag, keeping sleeve gathered.	____	____
11. Removed IV from pole. Slid bag and tubing through the sleeve. Kept bag above client's arm. Did not pull on the tubing. Placed used clothing on chair.	____	____
12. Hung bag back on the pole.	____	____
13. Gathered the sleeve of clean garment to be put on the arm with the IV.	____	____
14. Removed the IV bag from the pole. Made sure the bag is above the client's arm.	____	____
15. Slipped sleeve and garment shoulder over the bag. Placed bag back on the pole.	____	____
16. Slid the gathered sleeve over the tubing, hand, arm, and IV site.	____	____
17. Adjusted garment over client's shoulders and helped client to put other arm through other sleeve.	____	____
18. Checked that IV was working properly.	____	____
19. Assisted client to remove other garments and put on clean garments, as needed.	____	____
20. Made sure client was safe and comfortable.	____	____
21. Placed soiled garments in laundry container.	____	____
22. Placed bed in lowest position. (Raised side rail, if indicated.)*	____	____
23. Recorded what was done. Reported any abnormal conditions to supervisor.	____	____

Comments:

Evaluator's Signature: _____
Date: _____

*Will not apply if hospital bed is not used.

Procedure 14-15.   Helping With Range of Motion Exercises in Bed—General Procedure

Name: _____

	S	UN
1. Explained procedure to client.	___	___
2. Washed hands.	___	___
3. Provided privacy.	___	___
4. Raised bed to convenient working height. Lowered rail on side of bed.*	___	___
5. Folded top bedding to foot of bed. Covered client with sheet or blanket.	___	___
6. Helped client to move to side of bed near aide. Made sure client was in supine position.	___	___
7. Repeated each exercise as listed in the care plan.	___	___
8. Exercised upper body, both sides. Then exercised lower body, both sides.	___	___
9. Helped client to center of bed; replaced top bedding; removed sheet or blanket covering client.	___	___
10. Made sure client is safe and comfortable.	___	___
11. Placed bed in lowest position. (Raised side rail, if indicated.)*	___	___
12. Washed hands.	___	___
13. Recorded what was done. Reported any unusual conditions to supervisor or physical therapist.	___	___

SHOULDER/ARM EXERCISES

Held client's wrist and hand with one hand. With the other hand, grasped client's arm above the elbow.   ___ ___

    a. Moved arm, with palm down, forward and upward along side of head and downward to the side. Repeated with palm up.   ___ ___

    b. Moved arm with palm down, away from the body, sideways, to above the head and returned. Repeated with palm up.   ___ ___

FOREARM AND ELBOW EXERCISES

Rested client's upper arm on bed with forearm raised upright and elbow bent. Supported client's wrist and hand.   ___ ___

    a. Moved lower arm down, then up, with palm down. Repeated with palm up.   ___ ___

Rested client's upper arm on bed with forearm upright. Supported client's wrist with one hand and the client's hand with the other.   ___ ___

    a. Twisted palm toward client, then away.   ___ ___

WRIST EXERCISES

Held client's wrist with one hand and used other hand to perform movements: ___ ___

    a. Moved hand forward, then backward.   ___ ___

    b. Moved hand from one side to the other.   ___ ___

S   UN

FINGER EXERCISES
Held client's wrist with one hand. Used other hand to perform movements: ____ ____
    a. Bent fingers (made a fist), then straightened.   ____ ____
    b. Spread fingers and thumb apart, then brought together.   ____ ____

THUMB EXERCISES
Held client's hand and fingers with one hand. Used other hand to perform movements: ____ ____
    a. Moved thumb across palm of hand and straightened, then returned to side.   ____ ____
    b. Touched each finger tip with thumb.   ____ ____
    c. Bent thumb into palm and returned to straightened position.   ____ ____
    d. Moved thumb using wide, circular motion.   ____ ____

HIPS, LEG, AND KNEE EXERCISES
Supported client's leg with one hand under knee and other at the heel.   ____ ____
    a. Bent knee and raised toward chest, then lowered.   ____ ____
    b. Raised leg straight up as high as possible, then lowered leg gently.   ____ ____
Supported client's leg with one hand under knee and other hand under the ankle.   ____ ____
    a. Moved leg outward, away from body as far as possible. Returned to starting position.   ____ ____
    b. Moved leg across the other leg as far as possible and returned to starting position.   ____ ____
Placed one hand over top of knee and grasped. Placed other hand over top of ankle and grasped.   ____ ____
    a. Turned leg so toes are pointed inward, then outward.   ____ ____
Supported client's leg with one hand just above the knee and the other hand at the ankle.   ____ ____
    a. Bent the knee and slid the heel toward the buttocks as far as possible. Then straightened knee to starting position.   ____ ____

FOOT AND ANKLE EXERCISES
Supported ankle by placing client's heel in palm of one hand with other hand just above the ankle.   ____ ____
    a. Bent foot up toward the leg, then down, away from leg.   ____ ____
    b. Turned foot outward, sole facing away from body, then turned foot inward toward body.   ____ ____

TOE EXERCISES
Held client's foot with one hand. Used other hand to perform movements: ____ ____
    a. Bent toes down toward the ball of the foot, then bent toes back to front of foot.   ____ ____

Comments:

Evaluator's Signature: _____
Date: _____

Procedure 15-1.   Giving and Removing a Bedpan

Name: _____

	S	UN
1. Explained procedure to client.	____	____
2. Washed hands.	____	____
3. Obtained necessary materials.	____	____
4. Provided privacy.	____	____
5. Raised bed to convenient working height.*	____	____
6. Warmed bedpan with warm tap water. Dried with paper towels.	____	____
7. Took bedpan to bedside and placed on chair or bed.	____	____
8. Lowered rail on side of bed.*	____	____
9. Assisted client to lie on back. Elevated head of bed slightly.*	____	____
10. Folded back upper linens.	____	____
11. Instructed client to bend knees and raise buttocks. Assisted as needed. If bed or client was soiled, put on gloves.	____	____
12. Slid the bedpan under the client.	____	____
13. If the client could not raise the hips to get onto the bedpan, aide:	____	____
a. Turned the client on side, facing away from aide.	____	____
b. Positioned the bedpan firmly against the buttocks.	____	____
c. Turned the client onto back and held the bedpan in place under the buttocks.	____	____
14. Covered client with top sheet.	____	____
15. Raised side rail and placed bed in sitting position.*	____	____
16. Propped up client with pillows if the bed was not adjustable.	____	____
17. Made sure bedpan was in correct position.	____	____
18. Gave toilet paper and asked client to call when finished.	____	____
19. Left room. Removed gloves, if using. Discarded gloves.	____	____
20. Washed hands.	____	____
21. Returned to room when client called.	____	____
22. Lowered rail on side of bed.*	____	____
23. Put on gloves.	____	____
24. Placed client in flat position and removed bedpan in same manner used to give the bedpan.	____	____
25. Cleansed perineal area with toilet tissue if necessary, wiping from front to back.	____	____
26. Raised side rail.*	____	____
27. Covered bedpan, took to bathroom, and emptied contents. Measured output if necessary. Observed contents.	____	____
28. Rinsed bedpan with cold water, cleaned, and disinfected.	____	____
29. Removed and discarded gloves.	____	____
30. Washed hands.	____	____

S   UN

31. Put bedpan away.   ___ ___
32. Lowered rail on side of bed.*   ___ ___
33. Helped client to wash hands.   ___ ___
34. Made sure client was safe and comfortable.   ___ ___
35. Placed bed in lowest position. (Raised side rail, if indicated.)*   ___ ___
36. Washed hands.   ___ ___
37. Recorded what was done. Reported any abnormal elimination
     to supervisor.   ___ ___

Comments:

Evaluator's Signature: _____
Date: _____

*Will not apply if hospital bed is not used.

Procedure 15-2.   Giving and Removing a Urinal

Name: _____

	S	UN
1. Explained procedure to client	____	____
2. Washed hands.	____	____
3. Obtained necessary materials.	____	____
4. Provided privacy.	____	____
5. Took urinal to bedside and placed on chair or bed.	____	____
6. Assisted client to stand. If client could not stand, placed client on back.	____	____
7. Folded back upper linens.	____	____
8. Gave urinal to client so he could position it properly.	____	____
9. If client was unable to position urinal, put on gloves and positioned it for him.	____	____
10. Covered client with top sheet.	____	____
11. Left room. Removed gloves, if used. Discarded gloves.	____	____
12. Washed hands.	____	____
13. Returned to room when client called.	____	____
14. Put on gloves.	____	____
15. Removed urinal in the same manner it was given.	____	____
16. Covered urinal, took to bathroom, and emptied contents. Measured output if necessary. Observed urine.	____	____
17. Rinsed urinal with cold water, cleaned, and disinfected.	____	____
18. Removed and discarded gloves.	____	____
19. Washed hands.	____	____
20. Put urinal away.	____	____
21. Helped client to wash hands.	____	____
22. Made sure client was safe and comfortable.	____	____
23. Washed hands.	____	____
24. Recorded what was done. Reported any abnormal urine or urination to supervisor.	____	____

Comments:

Evaluator's Signature: _____
Date: _____

Procedure 15-3.   Measuring and Recording Intake and Output

Name: _____

	S	UN

INTAKE

1. Washed hands.
2. Obtained necessary materials.
3. Measured each remaining liquid separately after client finished eating or drinking. Poured into measuring cup.
4. Held at eye level and measured the amount left.
5. Subtracted the remaining amount from the amount of the original full serving.
6. Repeated for each liquid and recorded.
7. Rinsed, cleaned, dried, and stored container used to measure intake.
8. Washed hands.
9. Accurately recorded the amount of fluid intake and the time on the I & O form.

OUTPUT

1. Washed hands.
2. Put on gloves and other personal protective equipment as needed.
3. Emptied bedpan, urinal, commode pail, "hat," or emesis basin into a graduated container if original container was not marked for measuring.
4. Measured amount of liquid and discarded into toilet.
5. Rinsed, cleaned, disinfected, dried, and stored container used to measure output.
6. Removed and discarded gloves and other personal protective equipment.
7. Washed hands.
8. Accurately recorded the amount of fluid output and the time on the I & O form.
9. Reported any abnormal output to supervisor.

Comments:

Evaluator's Signature: _____
Date: _____

Procedure 15-4.   Care of the Client With an Indwelling Catheter

Name: _____

	S	UN
1. Explained procedure to client.	____	____
2. Washed hands.	____	____
3. Obtained necessary materials.	____	____
4. Provided privacy.	____	____
5. Put on gloves.	____	____
6. Performed perineal care.	____	____
7. Female client: Separated labia to visualize the urinary meatus. Male client: Retracted foreskin (if uncircumcised).	____	____
8. Moistened cotton balls or gauze with soap and water.	____	____
9. Washed catheter tube in a downward motion away from the urinary meatus for approximately 4 inches (20 cm). Used one cotton ball or gauze pad for each stroke. Rinsed with water in the same manner. Discarded used cotton balls or gauze into bag.	____	____
10. Taped and positioned catheter properly.	____	____
11. Removed waterproof protector pad. Replaced top linens.	____	____
12. Made sure client was safe and comfortable.	____	____
13. Cleaned materials and stored in proper location.	____	____
14. Removed and discarded gloves.	____	____
15. Washed hands.	____	____
16. Recorded what was done. Reported any abnormal conditions to supervisor.	____	____

Comments:

Evaluator's Signature: _____
Date: _____

Procedure 15-5.   Emptying a Catheter Drainage Bag

Name: _____

	S	UN
1. Explained procedure to client.	___	___
2. Washed hands.	___	___
3. Obtained necessary materials.	___	___
4. Provided privacy.	___	___
5. Put on gloves and other personal protective equipment, as needed.	___	___
6. Placed measuring container under drainage tube of collection bag.	___	___
7. Opened clamp on drainage tube so urine could empty into graduated container. The drainage tube did not touch the insides of the graduated container or any other surface.	___	___
8. Closed clamp and replaced drainage tube in the holder on collecting bag.	___	___
9. Measured urine, then discarded in toilet.	___	___
10. Rinsed, cleaned, disinfected, and stored graduate.	___	___
11. Removed and discarded gloves and other personal protective equipment.	___	___
12. Washed hands.	___	___
13. Recorded what was done. Reported any abnormal conditions to supervisor.	___	___

Comments:

Evaluator's Signature: _____

Date: _____

Procedure 15-6.   Applying a Condom Catheter

Name: _____

	S	UN
1. Explained procedure to client.	___	___
2. Washed hands.	___	___
3. Obtained necessary materials.	___	___
4. Provided privacy.	___	___
5. Helped client to lie on back.	___	___
6. Put on gloves.	___	___
7. Covered client with sheet or bath blanket as for perineal care.	___	___
8. If condom catheter was present, removed gently and placed in plastic bag.	___	___
9. Gave perineal care.	___	___
10. Attached collection bag to leg or bed frame.	___	___
11. Applied protective coating to the skin of the penis, if a self-adhesive catheter was used.	___	___
12. Held penis firmly. Rolled the condom catheter onto penis with drainage opening at the urinary meatus.	___	___
13. Secured edge of condom catheter in place with Velcro band. Was careful not to constrict the penis.	___	___
14. Connected catheter tip to drainage tubing.	___	___
15. Made sure tubing was in correct position and that tip of catheter was not twisted.	___	___
16. Made sure client was safe and comfortable.	___	___
17. Discarded used supplies in plastic bag.	___	___
18. Removed and discarded gloves.	___	___
19. Washed hands.	___	___
20. Recorded what was done. Reported any abnormal findings to supervisor.	___	___

Comments:

Evaluator's Signature: _____
Date: _____

Procedure 16-1.   Collecting a Routine Urine Specimen

Name: _____

	S	UN
1. Explained procedure to client.	___	___
2. Washed hands.	___	___
3. Obtained necessary materials.	___	___
4. Labeled container and placed in bathroom.	___	___
5. Put on gloves and other personal protective equipment, as needed.	___	___
6. Assisted client to bathroom or commode or offered bed pan or urinal.	___	___
7. Reminded client not to drop toilet paper into specimen. Asked client to discard paper into waste basket.	___	___
8. Had client void into commode, bedpan, urinal, or "hat."	___	___
9. Took bedpan/urinal or commode pail into bathroom.	___	___
10. Poured urine into graduate and then into specimen container until three-fourths full. Discarded remaining urine into toilet.	___	___
11. Put lid on specimen container.	___	___
12. Placed container into a plastic bag and then into a paper bag.	___	___
13. Cleaned materials and stored in proper location.	___	___
14. Removed and discarded gloves and other personal protective equipment.	___	___
15. Washed hands.	___	___
16. Helped client, as needed, back to bed, chair, etc	___	___
17. Stored specimen in refrigerator.	___	___
18. Recorded what was done. Reported any abnormal conditions to supervisor.	___	___

Comments:

Evaluator's Signature: _____
Date: _____

Procedure 16-2. Collecting a "Clean Catch" or Midstream Urine Specimen

Name: _____

	S	UN

1. Explained procedure to client. ____ ____
2. Washed hands. ____ ____
3. Obtained necessary materials. ____ ____
4. Opened kit. Removed contents and labeled container. ____ ____
5. Assisted client to bathroom or commode, or offered bedpan or urinal. ____ ____
6. Told client how to perform procedure. Instructed client to call when finished. ____ ____
7. If assistance was necessary, put on gloves. ____ ____
8. Gave perineal care using towelettes in specimen kit. ____ ____
9. Kept labia separated until specimen was collected so that urine did not flow over skin surfaces. In uncircumcised males, the foreskin was retracted until the specimen was collected. ____ ____
10. Collected the specimen ____ ____
   a. Asked client to begin voiding into urinal, bedpan, commode, or toilet. ____ ____
   b. Instructed client to stop voiding. ____ ____
   c. Held specimen container under urinary meatus, but did not allow it to touch the skin surface. Did not touch the inside of container with hands. ____ ____
   d. Asked client to restart voiding. ____ ____
   e. Caught enough urine to fill the container about halfway. ____ ____
   f. Asked client to stop voiding. ____ ____
   g. Removed container. ____ ____
   h. Instructed client to finish voiding. ____ ____
11. Put lid on specimen container. Was careful not to touch inside to keep the specimen clean. ____ ____
12. Placed container into a plastic bag and then into a paper bag. ____ ____
13. Assisted client to complete toileting, if necessary. ____ ____
14. Cleaned materials and stored in proper location. ____ ____
15. Removed and discarded gloves. ____ ____
16. Washed hands. ____ ____
17. Helped client, as needed, back to bed, chair, etc. ____ ____
18. Stored specimen in refrigerator. ____ ____
19. Recorded what was done. Reported any abnormal conditions to supervisor. ____ ____

Comments:

Evaluator's Signature: _____
Date: _____

Procedure 16-3.   Collecting a 24-Hour Urine Specimen

Name: _____

	S	UN
1. Explained procedure to client and family.	___	___
2. Washed hands.	___	___
3. Obtained necessary materials.	___	___
4. Labeled container.	___	___
5. Arranged urine container in bucket of ice in bathroom. Placed preservative in container, if needed.	___	___
6. Placed a sign saying "Save All Urine" in bathroom near toilet.	___	___
7. Put on gloves and other personal protective equipment, as needed.	___	___
8. Had client void first specimen. Discarded. Recorded time.	___	___
9. Removed and discarded gloves and other personal protective equipment after the first specimen and each time another specimen was handled. Discarded gloves and other personal protective equipment. Washed hands.	___	___
10. Collected all urine for the next 24 hours. Poured into specimen container.	___	___
11. Reminded client not to have bowel movement when urinating.	___	___
12. Recorded I & O if needed.	___	___
13. Added each urine specimen to the container immediately following voiding. Poured into graduated container using funnel, if needed and then into large container to avoid spilling and splashing.	___	___
14. Added ice to the bucket as necessary.	___	___
15. At the end of 24 hours, had client void as before. Placed final specimen in large container.	___	___
16. Recorded what was done. Reported any problems or abnormal conditions to supervisor.	___	___
17. Kept specimen on ice.	___	___
18. Dried container and placed in large plastic grocery bag for delivery to laboratory.	___	___

Comments:

Evaluator's Signature: _____

Date: _____

Procedure 16-4.   Straining Urine

Name: _____

	S	UN
1. Explained procedure to client and family.	____	____
2. Obtained necessary materials and placed in bathroom.	____	____
3. Placed sign saying "Strain All Urine" near toilet.	____	____
4. Washed hands.	____	____
5. Put on gloves (and goggles if needed).	____	____
6. Had client void into bedpan/urinal, commode, or urine collector (hat) in toilet.	____	____
7. Transferred urine into graduated container.	____	____
8. Placed strainer or gauze over specimen container.	____	____
9. Poured urine through strainer and into specimen container.	____	____
10. Inspected filter paper or gauze. If stones were present, wrapped them in the filter material and placed in the specimen container for transport to the laboratory. Labeled container. Stored in refrigerator.	____	____
11. If no stones were present, discarded urine. Discarded used disposable materials. Cleaned used reusable materials and prepared for reuse the next time the client voids.	____	____
12. Removed and discarded gloves. Removed goggles, if used.	____	____
13. Washed hands.	____	____
14. Recorded what was done. Reported any abnormal conditions to supervisor.	____	____

Comments:

Evaluator's Signature: _____
Date: _____

Procedure 16-5.   Collecting a Stool Specimen

Name: _____

	S	UN
1. Explained procedure to client.	___	___
2. Washed hands.	___	___
3. Obtained necessary materials.	___	___
4. Labeled container.	___	___
5. Assisted client to bathroom or commode or offered bedpan.	___	___
6. Asked client not to urinate, if possible, while having a bowel movement.	___	___
7. Put on gloves.	___	___
8. Transferred stool specimen container using tongue depressor and put on lid.	___	___
9. Flushed remaining feces down toilet and assisted client to complete toileting as necessary.	___	___
10. Removed and discarded gloves.	___	___
11. Washed hands.	___	___
12. Helped client, as needed, back to bed, chair, etc.	___	___
13. Stored specimen according to agency policy or supervisor's directions.	___	___
14. Recorded what was done. Reported any abnormal conditions to supervisor.	___	___

Comments:

Evaluator's Signature: _____
Date: _____

Procedure 16-6.   Collecting a Sputum Specimen

Name: _____

	S	**UN**
1. Explained procedure to client.	___	___
2. Washed hands.	___	___
3. Obtained necessary materials.	___	___
4. Labeled container.	___	___
5. Provided privacy.	___	___
6. Put on gloves (disposable mask, if needed).	___	___
7. Assisted client to rinse mouth with plain water.	___	___
8. Had client hold sputum specimen container in one hand, tissue in the other.	___	___
9. Instructed client to take a deep breath, hold if for a second, and then cough into tissue. Did not let client cough on aide. Had client repeat the coughing two or three times to loosen the sputum deep in the respiratory tract.	___	___
10. When client had loosened sputum, had client cough sputum directly into the specimen container.	___	___
11. Did not touch the inside of the container. Kept the outside clean and free of any sputum.	___	___
12. Put lid on specimen container.	___	___
13. Placed container into plastic bag, then into a paper bag.	___	___
14. Removed and discarded gloves (removed and discarded mask).	___	___
15. Washed hands.	___	___
16. Recorded what was done. Reported any abnormal conditions to supervisor.	___	___
17. Sent specimen to laboratory according to agency policy.	___	___

Comments:

Evaluator's Signature: _____
Date: _____

Procedure 17-1.   Cleaning a Thermometer (Glass or Oral Electronic)

Name: _____

	S	UN
1. Washed hands.	___	___
2. Obtained necessary materials.	___	___
3. Put on disposable gloves.	___	___
4. Wet cotton ball (or tissue) with soap and water.	___	___
5. Held thermometer by stem over sink or wastebasket.	___	___
6. Began at stem end. Washed from stem to bulb end, twisting cotton ball firmly.	___	___
7. Discarded used cotton ball.	___	___
8. Rinsed thermometer with a clean, wet cotton ball using the same twisting, downward movement.	___	___
9. Repeated washing and rinsing.	___	___
10. Dried with a tissue, wiping in the same downward movement.	___	___
11. Discarded tissue.	___	___
12. Stored thermometer properly.	___	___
13. Removed and discarded gloves. Washed hands.	___	___

Comments:

Evaluator's Signature: _____
Date: _____

Procedure 17-2. Taking an Oral Temperature (With Glass Thermometer)

Name: _____

	S	UN
1. Explained procedure to client. (Reminded client not to eat, drink, or smoke for 15 minutes.)	____	____
2. Had client lie down or rest in a chair.	____	____
3. Washed hands.	____	____
4. Obtained necessary materials.	____	____
5. Put on disposable gloves (optional).	____	____
6. Cleaned thermometer.	____	____
7. Shook down mercury to 95° F (35° C), if necessary.	____	____
8. Placed thermometer under client's tongue, as far back as possible, into either heat pocket.	____	____
9. Told client to keep mouth closed and not to talk.	____	____
10. Left thermometer in place for 3 minutes. (Took pulse and respirations at this time.)	____	____
11. Removed thermometer.	____	____
12. Wiped thermometer with tissue from stem end to bulb end. Discarded tissue. Did not touch any part of the thermometer that had been in client's mouth.	____	____
13. Read the thermometer and then placed it on a tissue.	____	____
14. Wrote the temperature (pulse and respirations) on the paper.	____	____
15. Cleaned and dried thermometer.	____	____
16. Shook down thermometer to 95° F (35° C).	____	____
17. Stored thermometer in holder in proper location.	____	____
18. Removed and discarded gloves (optional). Washed hands.	____	____
19. Recorded temperature on client record. Indicated (O) for oral temperature.	____	____
20. Reported any abnormal temperature to supervisor.	____	____

Comments:

Evaluator's Signature: _____
Date: _____

Procedure 17-3.   Taking an Oral Temperature (With Electronic Thermometer)

Name: _____

	S	UN
1. Explained procedure to client. (Reminded client not to eat, drink, or smoke for 15 minutes.)	____	____
2. Had client lie down or rest in a chair.	____	____
3. Washed hands.	____	____
4. Obtained necessary materials.	____	____
5. Put on disposable gloves (optional).	____	____
6. Cleaned thermometer.	____	____
7. Turned on thermometer.	____	____
8. Waited until it read "0" or showed "- - -" on the digital display window.	____	____
9. Placed thermometer under client's tongue, as far back as possible, into either heat pocket.	____	____
10. Told client to keep mouth closed and not to talk.	____	____
11. Left thermometer in place until it "beeped." (Took pulse and respirations at this time.)	____	____
12. Removed thermometer.	____	____
13. Wiped thermometer with tissue from stem end to bulb end. Discarded tissue. Did not touch any part of the thermometer that had been in client's mouth.	____	____
14. Read the thermometer and then placed it on a tissue.	____	____
15. Wrote the temperature (pulse and respirations) on the paper.	____	____
16. Cleaned and dried thermometer.	____	____
17. Turned off thermometer.	____	____
18. Stored thermometer in holder in proper location.	____	____
19. Removed and discarded gloves (optional). Washed hands.	____	____
20. Recorded temperature on client record. Indicated (O) for oral temperature.	____	____
21. Reported abnormal temperature to supervisor.	____	____

Comments:

Evaluator's Signature: _____
Date: _____

Procedure 17-4.   Taking an Oral Temperature (With a Single-Use Thermometer)

Name: _____

	S	UN
1. Explained procedure to client. (Reminded client not to eat, drink, or smoke for 15 minutes.)	____	____
2. Had client lie down or rest in a chair.	____	____
3. Washed hands.	____	____
4. Obtained necessary materials.	____	____
5. Removed thermometer from wapper.	____	____
6. Placed thermometer under client's tongue, as far back as possible, into either heat pocket.	____	____
7. Told client to keep mouth closed and not to talk.	____	____
8. Left thermometer in place for at least 1 minute. (Took pulse and respirations at this time.)	____	____
9. Removed thermometer. Did not touch any part of thermometer that has been in client's mouth. Waited 10 seconds and read the last colored dot on the thermometer. Placed the thermometer on a tissue.	____	____
10. Wrote the temperature on the paper.	____	____
11. Discarded thermometer.	____	____
12. Washed hands.	____	____
13. Recorded temperature on client record and indicated (O) for oral.	____	____
14. Reported abnormal temperature to supervisor.	____	____

Comments:

Evaluator's Signature: _____
Date: _____

Procedure 17-5.   Taking an Axillary Temperature

Name: _____

	S	UN
1. Explained procedure to client.	___	___
2. Had client lie down or sit down.	___	___
3. Washed hands.	___	___
4. Obtained necessary materials.	___	___
5. Cleaned thermometer, if glass or electronic.	___	___
6. Shook down mercury (glass thermometer) to 95° F (35° C) or turned on electronic thermometer. Or, removed single-use thermometer from wrapper.	___	___
7. Provided privacy.	___	___
8. Removed client's arm from sleeve. Exposed axilla.	___	___
9. Dried axilla with towel or washcloth. Placed thermometer in axilla so it is in contact with the skin.	___	___
10. Put client's arm across chest to hold thermometer in place. For infant or child, held arm in place as necessary.	___	___
11. Left thermometer in place:	___	___
Glass—10 minutes	___	___
Electronic—until "beep" was heard	___	___
Single use—3 minutes	___	___
(Took pulse and respirations at this time.)	___	___
12. Removed thermometer.	___	___
13. Wiped with tissue from stem end to bulb, if glass or electronic thermometer was used. Then discarded tissue.	___	___
14. Read thermometer and then placed it on a tissue.	___	___
15. Wrote the temperature on the paper.	___	___
16. Helped client put arm back in sleeve.	___	___
17. Turned off electronic thermometer, if used.	___	___
18. Cleaned and dried glass or electronic thermometer. Or discarded single-use thermometer.	___	___
19. Shook down glass thermometer, if used.	___	___
20. Stored thermometer in holder in proper location.	___	___
21. Washed hands.	___	___
22. Recorded temperature on client record. Indicated (A) for axillary temperature.	___	___
23. Reported abnormal temperature to supervisor.	___	___

Comments:

Evaluator's Signature: _____
Date: _____

Procedure 17-6.   Taking a Temperature (With Tympanic Thermometer)

Name: _____

	S	UN
1. Explained procedure to client.	___	___
2. Had client lie down or rest in a chair.	___	___
3. Provided privacy.	___	___
4. Washed hands.	___	___
5. Obtained necessary materials.	___	___
6. Asked client to turn head so ear was in front of aide.	___	___
7. Pulled top of ear up and back to straighten the ear canal (in adults); or, pulled ear lobe down and back in a child under 2 years.	___	___
8. Gently inserted tympanic thermometer probe with cover into the ear canal.	___	___
9. Read the measurement when flashing light was seen or tone heard.	___	___
10. Removed thermometer probe from ear canal.	___	___
11. Discarded probe cover directly into the wastebasket.	___	___
12. Wrote the temperature on the paper. Indicated (T) for tympanic temperature.	___	___
13. Returned thermometer to base unit for recharge.	___	___
14. Washed hands.	___	___
15. Recorded what was done. Reported abnormal temperature to supervisor.	___	___

Comments:

Evaluator's Signature: _____
Date: _____

Procedure 17-7.   Taking a Rectal Temperature

Name: _____

	S	UN
1. Explained procedure to client.	____	____
2. Put client in bed.	____	____
3. Washed hands.	____	____
4. Obtained necessary materials.	____	____
5. Cleaned glass thermometer.	____	____
6. Shook down mercury in glass thermometer to 95° F (35° C), if necessary.	____	____
7. Provided privacy.	____	____
8. Placed client in Sims' position.	____	____
9. Put on gloves.	____	____
10. Placed small amount of lubricant on toilet tissue. Lubricated bulb end of thermometer.	____	____
11. Folded back top linens and removed clothing to expose anal area.	____	____
12. Raised upper buttock to expose anus.	____	____
13. Gently inserted thermometer 1 inch (2.5 cm) into the rectum.	____	____
14. Held in place for 3 minutes.	____	____
15. Removed thermometer.	____	____
16. Wiped thermometer with toilet tissue from stem end to bulb end. Placed soiled tissue on several folded layers of toilet tissue.	____	____
17. Placed thermometer on clean toilet tissue.	____	____
18. Cleansed excess lubricant and feces from anal area using toilet tissue.	____	____
19. Replaced clothing and covered client.	____	____
20. Discarded soiled toilet tissue into toilet.	____	____
21. Removed and discarded gloves. Washed hands.	____	____
22. Read the thermometer and then placed it back on tissue.	____	____
23. Wrote the temperature on the paper.	____	____
24. Cleaned and dried glass thermometer. Discarded single-use thermometer.	____	____
25. Shook down glass thermometer to 95° F (35° C).	____	____
26. Stored thermometer in holder in proper location.	____	____
27. Washed hands.	____	____
28. Made sure client was safe and comfortable.	____	____
29. Recorded temperature on client record. Indicated (R) for rectal temperature.	____	____
30. Reported abnormal temperature to supervisor.	____	____

Comments:

Evaluator's Signature: _____
Date: _____

Procedure 17-8.   Taking a Radial Pulse

Name: _____

	S	UN
1. Explained procedure to client.	____	____
2. Asked client to sit or lie down.	____	____
3. Washed hands.	____	____
4. Obtained necessary materials.	____	____
5. Located radial pulse. Used middle three fingers to press down on radial artery.	____	____
6. Noted the following:	____	____
Strong or weak	____	____
Regular or irregular	____	____
7. Counted the beats for 1 minute.	____	____
8. Wrote the pulse rate on the paper. Also noted the strength and regularity of beats.	____	____
9. Made sure client was safe and comfortable.	____	____
10. Recorded pulse on client record.	____	____
11. Reported any abnormal pulse conditions to supervisor.	____	____

Comments:

Evaluator's Signature: _____
Date: _____

Procedure 17-9. Taking Respirations

Name: _____

	S	UN
1. Continued holding client's wrist after taking the pulse.	____	____
2. Did not tell the client that respirations were going to be counted.	____	____
3. Counted each rise and fall of the chest or abdomen as one respiration.	____	____
4. Counted respirations for 1 minute.	____	____
5. Observed for the following:	____	____
Deep or shallow breathing	____	____
Painful or difficulty breathing	____	____
Noisy breathing	____	____
6. Recorded respirations on paper, noted information listed above.	____	____
7. Made sure client was safe and comfortable.	____	____
8. Washed hands.	____	____
9. Recorded respirations on client record.	____	____
10. Reported any abnormal respirations to supervisor.	____	____

Comments:

Evaluator's Signature: _____
Date: _____

Procedure 17-10. Measuring Blood Pressure

Name: _____

	S	**UN**
1. Explained procedure to client.	___	___
2. Asked client to sit or lie down.	___	___
3. Washed hands.	___	___
4. Obtained necessary materials.	___	___
5. Wiped stethoscope earpieces and chest piece (diaphragm) or bell with antiseptic wipes.	___	___
6. Placed client's arm in position level with the heart, palm up, supported by a pillow(s), table, or arm of chair.	___	___
7. Exposed the client's upper arm. Removed clothing so that area was bare.	___	___
8. Squeezed the blood pressure cuff to expel any air. Closed the valve of the bulb.	___	___
9. Found the brachial artery by feeling the pulse at the inner side of the elbow.	___	___
10. Wrapped the cuff around the client's arm, at least 1 inch above the bend in the arm. Made sure cuff was secure and even. Positioned rubber bag over the artery.	___	___
11. Put stethoscope ear pieces in ears.	___	___
12. Placed fingers over radial pulse. Inflated the cuff until radial pulse could not be felt. Inflated the cuff 30 mm beyond the point at which the pulse was last felt.	___	___
13. Placed stethoscope chest piece (diaphragm) or bell over the brachial artery.	___	___
14. Kept eyes on dial and began to deflate the cuff slowly and evenly (2 to 4 millimeters per second) by turning the valve of the bulb counterclockwise.	___	___
15. Noted the first sound heard and read the dial at that point.	___	___
16. Kept eyes on dial and continued to deflate the cuff. Noted the last sound heard and read the dial at that point.	___	___
17. Deflated the cuff completely. Removed the stethoscope and cuff from the client's arm.	___	___
18. Wrote the blood pressure measurement on the paper.	___	___
19. Assisted client, as needed, to desired position.	___	___
20. Cleaned earpieces and chest piece (diaphragm) or bell of stethoscope with antiseptic wipes. Discarded used wipes.	___	___
21. Returned all materials to proper storage place.	___	___
22. Washed hands.	___	___
23. Recorded accurate blood pressure on client record.	___	___
24. Reported blood pressure that was above or below normal to supervisor.	___	___

Comments:

Evaluator's Signature: _____

Date: _____

Procedure 18-1.   Assisting With Oral Medications

Name: _____

	S	UN
1. Explained procedure to client.	___	___
2. Checked care plan and medication sheet.	___	___
3. Washed hands.	___	___
4. Obtained necessary materials.	___	___
5. Helped client to wash hands.	___	___
6. Checked label on each prescription or on each prepoured medication for:	___	___

Right Drug   Right Dose   Right Time
Right Client   Right Route

7. Loosened lid(s) on the container(s) if client was unable to do so. Told client name of each medication (read from label).   ___ ___
8. Placed containers where client could reach them or handed containers to client. Let client read name of medication to aide. Made sure client was wearing eyeglasses if needed.   ___ ___
9. Assisted client with oral medications: ___ ___
Gave sip of water to moisten mouth.   ___ ___
Supported hand as necessary to pour medication.   ___ ___
Gave a full glass of water or other cool liquid after client put medication in mouth.   ___ ___
Reminded client to lower chin while swallowing.   ___ ___
10. Closed containers.   ___ ___
11. Had client record medication(s) taken. (Aide recorded, if necessary.)   ___ ___
12. Stored materials in proper location.   ___ ___
13. Washed hands.   ___ ___
14. Recorded what was done. Reported any abnormal conditions to supervisor.   ___ ___

Comments:

Evaluator's Signature: _____

Date: _____

Procedure 18-2.   Assisting With Rectal Suppositories

Name: _____

	S	UN
1. Explained procedure to client.	___	___
2. Checked care plan and medication sheet.	___	___
3. Washed hands.	___	___
4. Obtained necessary materials.	___	___
5. Provided privacy.	___	___
6. Assisted client into bed and Sims' position.	___	___
7. Removed clothing to expose anal area.	___	___
8. Checked label on the suppository for:	___	___

Right Drug   Right Dose   Right Time
Right Client   Right Route

	S	UN
9. Unwrapped suppository.	___	___
10. Applied water-soluble lubricant to suppository.	___	___
11. Gave glove to client to put on.	___	___
12. Handed suppository to client to insert into rectum. Guided client's hand, if necessary.	___	___
13. Observed as client inserted medication and wiped anus with toilet tissue.	___	___
14. Had client remove and discard glove into waste container.	___	___
15. Assisted client to wash hands.	___	___
16. Discarded used materials in waste container.	___	___
17. Had client record medication(s) taken. (Aide recorded for client, if necessary.)	___	___
18. Reminded client to remain on side for 15 to 20 minutes to allow suppository to melt and medication to be absorbed.	___	___
19. Washed hands.	___	___
20. Recorded what was done. Reported any abnormal conditions to supervisor.	___	___

Comments:

Evaluator's Signature: _____

Date: _____

Procedure 18-3.   Assisting With Eye Medications or Ointment

Name: _____

	S	UN
1. Explained procedure to client.	___	___
2. Checked care plan and medication sheet.	___	___
3. Washed hands. Put on disposable gloves (optional).	___	___
4. Obtained necessary materials.	___	___
5. Helped client to wash hands.	___	___
6. Checked label on prescription container for:	___	___

6. Checked label on prescription container for:

Right Drug—was certain the preparation was for use in the eyes only   ___ ___
Right Client   ___ ___
Right Dose—was certain the strength of the solution/ointment in   ___ ___
the container was correct
Right Route—which eye, or both eyes   ___ ___
Right Time

7. Loosened lid on container, if client was unable to do so.   ___ ___
8. Placed container within client's reach or handed to client as necessary.   ___ ___
   Made sure client was wearing eyeglasses, if needed.   ___ ___
9. Held mirror so client could see to administer eye medication.   ___ ___
10. Removed client's eyeglasses, if worn.   ___ ___
11. Assisted client with: ___ ___

EYE MEDICATIONS

Guided client's hand to grasp lower lid.   ___ ___
Observed that client looked up and released drops into lower lid.   ___ ___
Observed that client closed eye to distribute medication   ___ ___
Made sure that dropper did not touch client's eye.   ___ ___

EYE OINTMENT

Guided client's hand to grasp lower lid.   ___ ___
Observed that client looked up and squeezed a small ribbon of ointment   ___ ___
into the lower lid from inner corner of eye to outer corner of eye.
Observed that client closed eye to allow medication to melt and be   ___ ___
distributed. Made sure that tip of tube did not touch eye surface.
12. Resealed container.   ___ ___
13. Had client record medication(s) taken. (Aide recorded for client, if   ___ ___
   necessary.)
14. Stored materials in proper location.   ___ ___
15. Removed and discarded gloves (optional). Washed hands.   ___ ___
16. Recorded what was done. Reported any abnormal conditions to supervisor.   ___ ___

Comments:

Evaluator's Signature: _____
Date: _____

Procedure 18-4.   Assisting With Transdermal Disks

Name: _____

	S	UN
1. Explained procedure to client.	___	___
2. Checked care plan and medication sheet.	___	___
3. Washed hands. Put on gloves (optional).	___	___
4. Obtained necessary materials.	___	___
5. Provided privacy.	___	___
6. Helped client to wash hands.	___	___
7. Checked label on disk container for:	___	___

Right Drug   Right Dose   Right Time
Right Client   Right Route

8. Had client remove and discard old disk into waste container. Washed skin that had been covered by old disk.	___	___
9. Asked client to select new site for new disk (any area without hair), usually the chest or upper arm.	___	___
10. Observed as client applied new disk to skin surface. Aide did not touch medicated surface of disk with ungloved fingers.	___	___
11. Discarded disk wrapper and other used materials.	___	___
12. Had client record medication(s) taken. (Aide recorded for client, if necessary.)	___	___
13. Stored materials in proper location.	___	___
14. Removed and discarded gloves (optional). Washed hands.	___	___
15. Recorded what was done. Reported any abnormal conditions to supervisor.	___	___

Comments:

Evaluator's Signature: _____
Date: _____

Procedure 18-5.   Assisting With Metered-Dose Inhalers

Name: _____

	S	UN
1. Explained procedure to client.	____	____
2. Checked care plan and medication sheet.	____	____
3. Washed hands.	____	____
4. Obtained necessary materials.	____	____
5. Provided privacy.	____	____
6. Helped client to wash hands.	____	____
7. Checked label on prescription container for:	____	____

Right Drug   Right Dose   Right Time
Right Client   Right Route

	S	UN
8. Handed metered-dose inhaler to client, who then used it to inhale medication.	____	____
9. Had client record medication taken. (Aide recorded for client, if necessary.)	____	____
10. Cleaned inhaler, wearing disposable gloves, according to manufacturer's instructions and stored in proper location.	____	____
11. Removed and discarded gloves. Washed hands.	____	____
12. Recorded what was done. Reported any abnormal conditions to supervisor.	____	____
13. Assisted client with oral hygiene, as needed.	____	____

Comments:

Evaluator's Signature: _____
Date: _____

Procedure 18-6.   Applying a Hot Water Bag

Name: _____

	S	UN

1. Explained procedure to client.
2. Washed hands.
3. Obtained necessary materials.
4. Provided privacy.
5. Filled hot water bag with water. Secured with stopper. Turned bag upside down to check for leaks.
6. Removed stopper and emptied bag.
7. Ran more hot water and tested with cooking thermometer; adjusted water temperature to 115°-130° F or 46°-54.4° C.
8. Filled bag one-third to one-half full.
9. Laid bag flat to remove air. Placed stopper in bag while it was still flat.
10. Covered bag with soft cloth or towel and applied to client's affected area.
11. Wrote the time the bag was applied.
12. Refilled bag when it became cool.
13. Checked client's skin every 10 minutes for danger signs.
14. Removed bag according to time required. Wrote time of removal on paper.
15. Removed stopper, emptied bag, and hung bag upside down to dry. Placed cloth or towel in laundry container.
16. Washed hands.
17. Recorded what was done. Reported any unusual conditions to supervisor.
18. When bag was dry, blew air into it and replaced stopper to prevent inside of bag from sticking together. Stored in proper location.

Comments:

Evaluator's Signature: _____
Date: _____

Procedure 18-7.   Applying a Hot/Cold Pack

Name: _____

	S	UN
1. Explained procedure to client.	____	____
2. Washed hands.	____	____
3. Obtained necessary materials.	____	____
4. Provided privacy.	____	____
5. Placed hot pack in microwave and heated according to manufacturer's directions. Or, removed cold pack from freezer.	____	____
6. Covered pack with soft cloth, towel, or cover and applied to client's affected area.	____	____
7. Wrote the time pack was applied.	____	____
8. Checked client's skin every 10 minutes for danger signs.	____	____
9. Removed pack according to time required. Wrote time of removal on paper.	____	____
10. Stored pack according to manufacturer's directions. Placed cloth, towel, or cover in laundry container.	____	____
11. Washed hands.	____	____
12. Recorded what was done. Reported any unusual conditions to supervisor.	____	____

Comments:

Evaluator's Signature: _____

Date: _____

Procedure 18-8.   Applying Hot Compresses

Name: _____

	S	UN
1. Explained procedure to client.	___	___
2. Washed hands.	___	___
3. Obtained necessary materials.	___	___
4. Provided privacy.	___	___
5. Placed waterproof protector pad under the body part where compress will be applied.	___	___
6. Filled basin or container one-half to two-thirds full of water at 105°-115° F (40.5°-46.1° C). Checked temperature with cooking thermometer.	___	___
7. Put on gloves.	___	___
8. Placed compress in the water.	___	___
9. Wrung out compress and applied to area. Noted time applied.	___	___
10. Covered compress quickly with plastic wrap. Secured edges of plastic wrap with tape. Covered with bath towel.	___	___
11. Wrote the time compress was applied.	___	___
12. Applied, according to directions, a hot water bag or rubber-protected heating pad over the plastic wrap to keep compress hot.	___	___
13. Checked client's skin every 10 minutes for danger signs.	___	___
14. Changed compress, if cooling occurred.	___	___
15. Removed compress according to time required.	___	___
16. Wrote time of removal on paper.	___	___
17. Patted area dry with towel. Discarded used compress. Placed used cloths or towels in laundry container.	___	___
18. Removed and discarded gloves.	___	___
19. Washed hands.	___	___
20. Cleaned and stored materials in proper location.	___	___
21. Recorded what was done. Reported any unusual conditions to supervisor.	___	___

Comments:

Evaluator's Signature: ____   _____
Date: _____

Procedure 18-9.   Applying Hot Soaks

Name: _____

	S	UN
1. Explained procedure to client.	___	___
2. Washed hands.	___	___
3. Obtained necessary materials.	___	___
4. Provided privacy.	___	___
5. Assisted client to comfortable position.	___	___
6. Placed waterproof protector pad under the area to be soaked.	___	___
7. Filled basin or container one-half full of water 105°-110° F (40.5°-43.3° C). Checked temperature with cooking thermometer.	___	___
8. Exposed only the part to be soaked.	___	___
9. Placed area to be soaked into the water.	___	___
10. Checked water temperature and skin of area being soaked every 10 minutes. Removed from water if danger signs were noticed.	___	___
11. Removed body part from water according to time required.	___	___
12. Wrote time of removal.	___	___
13. Patted body part dry. Assisted client to replace clothing and to get comfortable.	___	___
14. Cleaned and stored materials in proper location.	___	___
15. Put used towel in laundry container.	___	___
16. Washed hands.	___	___
17. Recorded what was done. Reported any unusual conditions to supervisor.	___	___

Comments:

Evaluator's Signature: _____

Date: _____

Procedure 18-10.   Giving a Sitz Bath

Name: _____

	S	UN
1. Explained procedure to client.	___	___
2. Washed hands.	___	___
3. Obtained necessary materials.	___	___
4. Assisted client to bathroom or commode.	___	___
5. Provided privacy.	___	___
6. Put on gloves.	___	___
7. Helped client to remove clothing from below waist.	___	___
8. Asked client to remove and discard dressing or pad, if worn. Assisted, if needed. Observed amount and color of drainage.	___	___
9. Asked client to void before beginning the procedure.	___	___
10. Raised toilet seat. Placed sitz bowl so that drainage holes were at the back of the toilet. Filled half of plastic sitz bowl with warm water, 94°-98° F (34°-37° C). Checked temperature with cooking thermometer.	___	___
11. Closed side clamp of bag tubing. Filled water bag with warm water, 120° F (49° C). Hung bag so that it was higher than the toilet (on towel bar, top of toilet tank, or vanity).	___	___
12. Assisted client to sit in sitz bowl. If client felt cold, covered shoulders and knees with blanket or towel.	___	___
13. Placed tube end of water bag in outlet at front of the bowl.	___	___
14. Instructed client to open clamp of water bag to let warmer water into the bowl when water began to cool. Assisted as needed.	___	___
15. Instructed client to call for assistance, if needed. Explained that the procedure will take 15 to 20 minutes.	___	___
16. Removed and discarded gloves.	___	___
17. Washed hands.	___	___
18. Checked client's condition every 7 minutes or more frequently, if needed.	___	___
19. When time was up, clamped tubing and removed from sitz bath.	___	___
20. Washed hands. Put on second pair of gloves.	___	___
21. Assisted client to slowly assume standing position.	___	___
22. Inspected perineal area; noted any drainage in water. Dried area and reapplied dressing or pad, if needed.	___	___
23. Assisted client to dress, as needed, and returned to bed or chair.	___	___
24. Emptied and disinfected plastic bowl. Flushed tubing with warm water and cleaned end of tubing. Returned equipment to proper location.	___	___
25. Removed and discarded gloves.	___	___
26. Washed hands.	___	___
27. Straightened bathroom.	___	___
28. Recorded on care record; noted color and amount of drainage on dressing or pad. Reported any unusual conditions to supervisor.	___	___

Comments:

Evaluator's Signature: _____

Date: _____

Procedure 18-11.   Applying an Ice Bag

Name: _____

	S	UN
1. Explained procedure to client.	____	____
2. Washed hands.	____	____
3. Obtained materials listed above.	____	____
4. Provided privacy.	____	____
5. Filled ice bag with water. Secured with stopper. Turned bag upside down to check for leaks.	____	____
6. Removed stopper and emptied bag.	____	____
7. Crushed the ice and filled bag (one-half to two-thirds full).	____	____
8. Laid bag flat to remove air. Placed stopper in bag while it was still flat.	____	____
9. Covered bag with soft cloth or towel and applied to client's affected area.	____	____
10. Wrote on paper the time the bag was applied.	____	____
11. Added ice as bag warmed. Changed towel if it became moist.	____	____
12. Checked client's skin every 10 minutes for danger signs.	____	____
13. Removed bag according to time required. Wrote time of removal.	____	____
14. Removed stopper, emptied bag, and placed bag upside down to dry. Placed cloth or towel in laundry container to be washed.	____	____
15. Washed hands.	____	____
16. Recorded what was done. Reported any unusual conditions to supervisor.	____	____
17. When bag was dry, blew air into it and replaced stopper to prevent insides of bag from sticking together. Stored in proper location.	____	____

Comments:

Evaluator's Signature: _____
Date: _____

Procedure 18-12.   Applying Cold Compresses

Name: _____

	S	UN
1. Explained procedure to client.	___	___
2. Washed hands.	___	___
3. Obtained necessary materials.	___	___
4. Provided privacy.	___	___
5. Placed waterproof protector pad under the body part where compress is to be applied.	___	___
6. Filled basin or container one-half to two-thirds full with ice water.	___	___
7. Put on gloves.	___	___
8. Placed compress in water.	___	___
9. Wrung out compress and applied to area.	___	___
10. Covered compress quickly with plastic wrap. Secured edges of plastic wrap with tape. Covered with bath towel.	___	___
11. Recorded the time the compress was applied.	___	___
12. Checked client's skin every 10 minutes for danger signs.	___	___
13. Changed compress when warming occurred.	___	___
14. Removed compress according to time required.	___	___
15. Wrote time of removal.	___	___
16. Patted area dry with towel. Discarded used gauze square or compresses. Placed used cloths and towels in laundry container.	___	___
17. Removed and discarded gloves.	___	___
18. Washed hands.	___	___
19. Cleaned and stored materials in proper location.	___	___
20. Recorded what was done. Reported any unusual conditions to supervisor.	___	___

Comments:

Evaluator's Signature: _____
Date: _____

Procedure 18-13.   Removing a Soiled Dressing and Applying a Clean, Dry Dressing

Name: _____

	S	UN

1. Explained procedure to client.
2. Washed hands.
3. Obtained necessary materials.
4. Provided privacy.
5. Cut lengths of tapes needed and hung them on edge of table for later use.
6. Put on gloves.

REMOVING SOILED DRESSING

7. Exposed area where dressing was to be removed.
8. Placed paper or plastic bag nearby.
9. Removed all tape from skin by pulling tape toward the dressing/wound.
10. Gently removed soiled dressing using tongs or clothespin to grasp the edges. If tongs or clothespin were not available, grasped the cleanest part of the dressing and removed. Inspected dressing and skin. Noted color, amount of drainage, and odor. Discarded into paper bag.
11. Discarded soiled gloves, washed hands. Put on clean gloves.

APPLYING CLEAN, DRY DRESSING

12. Removed clean, dry dressing from cover, touching the edge of dressing only.
13. Applied dressing to area.
14. Took strips of precut tape and applied to secure dressing.
15. Placed dressing cover in paper bag and discarded.
16. Removed and discarded gloves in paper or plastic bag.
17. Washed hands.
18. Recorded what was done. Reported any unusual conditions to supervisor.

Comments:

Evaluator's Signature: _____
Date: _____

Procedure 18-14.   Applying Elastic Stockings

Name: _____

		S	UN
1.	Explained procedure to client.	____	____
2.	Washed hands.	____	____
3.	Obtained elastic stockings.	____	____
4.	Provided privacy.	____	____
5.	Placed client in supine position.	____	____
6.	Exposed legs. Checked to see that legs were clean and dry.	____	____
7.	Turned stocking inside out by placing one hand into sock, holding toe of sock with other hand, and pulling.	____	____
8.	Placed client's toes into foot of stocking. Made sure sock was smooth.	____	____
9.	Slid remaining portion of sock over client's foot and heel. Made sure foot fit into toe and heel position of the sock. (The sock is now right side out.)	____	____
10.	Pulled stocking up over client's calf until stocking was fully extended.	____	____
11.	Inspected stocking to make sure there were no wrinkles or binding at top of stocking.	____	____
12.	Made sure client was safe and comfortable.	____	____
13.	Washed hands.	____	____
14.	Recorded what was done. Reported any unusual conditions to supervisor.	____	____
15.	Checked circulation regularly according to care plan.	____	____

Comments:

Evaluator's Signature: _____
Date: _____

Procedure 18-15.   Applying Elastic Bandages

Name: _____

	S	UN
1. Explained procedure to client.	___	___
2. Washed hands.	___	___
3. Obtained necessary materials.	___	___
4. Provided privacy.	___	___
5. Assisted client to comfortable position—supine for legs and feet; other positions according to care plan and part to be bandaged.	___	___
6. Exposed part. Checked to see that it was clean and dry.	___	___
7. Held the bandage with roll up.	___	___
8. Applied one end of bandage to the smallest part (e.g., wrist, ankle).	___	___
9. Wrapped two turns to anchor bandage.	___	___
10. Continued wrapping in spiral turns upward (overlapped previous turn by two thirds). Applied firmly but NOT TOO TIGHTLY.	___	___
11. Fastened end with clip, pin, or tape.	___	___
12. Washed hands.	___	___
13. Recorded what was done. Reported any unusual conditions to supervisor.	___	___
14. Checked for proper circulation regularly according to care plan.	___	___

Comments:

Evaluator's Signature: _____
Date: _____

Procedure 20-1.   Bathing an Infant—Sponge Bath

Name: _____

	S	UN
1. Washed hands.	___	___
2. Obtained necessary materials.	___	___
3. Placed all materials in easy reach. Spread hooded towel or receiving blanket on flat surface near where baby will be bathed.	___	___
4. Placed baby on receiving blanket or hooded towel next to basin of warm water. Always kept one hand on baby. Never left baby unattended.	___	___
5. Began with the head:	___	___
a. Wet a cotton ball with plain water and gently cleaned eye by wiping from inner corner to outer corner. Discarded cotton ball. Used a new one to clean other eye.	___	___
b. Wet washcloth and sponged face, ears, and folds in neck. Patted dry.	___	___
c. Picked up baby, holding in the football hold, facing upright. Held head over basin. With free hand, wet washcloth and wrung out over baby's scalp. Put a small amount of soap on the palm of hand. Rubbed gently on to the infant's scalp. Rinsed by wringing wet washcloth over head. Dried gently. Covered head with hooded towel or receiving blanket.	___	___
6. Removed shirt. Washed chest, upper abdomen, arms, and hands. Patted dry. Turned baby, washed and dried back.	___	___
7. Put on clean shirt.	___	___
8. Cleaned umbilical cord with alcohol (according to care plan).	___	___
9. Removed lower clothing. Washed legs and feet and dried.	___	___
10. Put on gloves.	___	___
11. Removed diaper. Wiped any feces away with tissue and cleaned perineal area. Discarded diaper or set aside for laundry. Washed perineum:	___	___
a. Girls—washed from front to back, rinsed thoroughly. Gently patted dry.	___	___
b. Boys—washed entire scrotum. Cared for circumcision according to care plan.	___	___
12. Put on dry diaper.	___	___
13. Removed and discarded gloves.	___	___
14. Finished dressing baby. Wrapped in receiving blanket.	___	___
15. Placed baby in a safe and comfortable position.	___	___
16. Cleaned materials and returned to proper location.	___	___
17. Recorded what was done. Reported any unusual observations to supervisor.	___	___

Comments:

Evaluator's Signature: _____

Date: _____

Procedure 20-2.   Bathing an Infant—Tub Bath

Name: _____

	S	UN
1. Washed hands.	___	___
2. Obtained necessary materials.	___	___
3. Placed all materials in easy reach. Spread hooded towel or receiving blanket on flat surface near where baby will be bathed.	___	___
4. Placed baby on receiving blanket or hooded towel next to basin of warm water. Always kept one hand on baby. Never left baby unattended.	___	___
5. Began with the head:	___	___
a. Wet a cotton ball with plain water and gently cleaned eye by wiping from inner corner to outer corner. Discarded cotton ball. Used a new one to clean other eye.	___	___
b. Wet washcloth and sponged face, ears, and folds in neck. Patted dry.	___	___
c. Picked up baby, holding in the football hold, facing upright. Held head over basin. With free hand, wet washcloth and wrung out over baby's scalp. Put a small amount of soap on the palm of hand. Rubbed gently on to the infant's scalp. Rinsed by wringing wet washcloth over head. Dried gently. Covered head with hooded towel or receiving blanket.	___	___
6. Laid baby back on flat surface.	___	___
7. Removed shirt.	___	___
8. Put on gloves.	___	___
9. Removed diaper. Wiped any feces away with tissue and cleaned perineal area. Discarded diaper or set aside for laundry.	___	___
10. Removed and discarded gloves.	___	___
11. Held infant:	___	___
a. Placed left hand under baby's shoulders. Thumb was over the baby's left shoulder. Aide's hand held the upper left arm.	___	___
b. Used right hand to support the baby's buttocks. Slid hand under the thigh. Held left thigh with right hand.	___	___
12. Lowered baby in water, feet first.	___	___
13. Washed front of infant's body, using right hand.	___	___
14. Changed hold:	___	___
a. Used right hand to support baby in a sitting forward position.	___	___
b. Supported and held fingers around baby's upper arm and placed hand under the infant's chin, as in lap position for burping.	___	___
15. Washed baby's back.	___	___
16. Returned to previous position.	___	___
17. Washed genital area.	___	___
18. Lifted baby out of water and onto towel.	___	___
19. Wrapped baby in towel, covered head.	___	___

	S	UN
20. Patted baby dry.	____	____
21. Put on dry diaper.	____	____
22. Finished dressing baby. Wrapped in receiving blanket.	____	____
23. Placed baby in safe and comfortable position.	____	____
24. Cleaned materials and returned to proper location.	____	____
25. Recorded what was done. Reported any unusual observations to supervisor.	____	____

Comments:

Evaluator's Signature: _____
Date: _____

Procedure 20-3. Dressing an Infant

Name: _____

	S	UN

1. Applied shirt:
   a. Stretched neck of shirt and pulled over baby's head.
   b. Placed hand inside sleeve and reached up through sleeve to grasp baby's hand and pulled through.
   c. Repeated on other side.
   d. Pulled shirt down over chest. If umbilical stump is present, folded bottom of shirt up to avoid rubbing.
2. Applied one piece sleeper:
   a. Unfastened all snaps on sleeper.
   b. Laid garment on flat surface.
   c. Placed baby on garment.
   d. Inserted feet into lower portion of sleeper.
   e. Reached through sleeves (as for shirts) to put on upper portion of sleeper.
   f. Snapped up garment.
3. Applied booties:
   a. Rolled bootie over hand, inside out.
   b. Grasped infant's toes and turned bootie up and over foot with other hand.

Comments:

Evaluator's Signature: _____
Date: _____

Procedure 20-4.   Changing a Diaper

Name: _____

	S	UN
1. Washed hands.	____	____
2. Obtained necessary materials	____	____
3. Put on gloves.	____	____
4. Placed baby on changing surface near materials. Made sure to protect baby from rolling off surface.	____	____
5. Opened soiled diaper.	____	____
6. Wiped genital area with front of diaper (if dry). Wiped from front to back.	____	____
7. Rolled diaper so that urine and feces are inside. Set aside for later disposal.	____	____
8. Washed the perineal area with soap and water or used baby wipes. Rinsed and dried thoroughly.	____	____
9. Gave cord/circumcision care according to care plan.	____	____
10. Raised baby's legs. Placed clean diaper in place. Cloth diaper was folded to better fit baby.	____	____
a. Girls—extra fold in back.	____	____
b. Boys—extra fold in front.	____	____
11. Pinned or fastened diaper in place. Kept diaper below umbilical stump. Was careful not to stick baby with diaper pin. Had finger under diaper when pin was inserted.	____	____
12. Applied plastic pants (if cloth diaper was used).	____	____
13. Placed baby in safe and comfortable position.	____	____
14. Rinsed (or dumped) feces from diaper into toilet. Flushed. Rinsed cloth diaper with cool water and placed in diaper pail for laundering. Discarded disposable diaper in garbage.	____	____
15. Removed and discarded gloves.	____	____
16. Washed hands.	____	____
17. Recorded what was done. Reported any unusual observations to supervisor.	____	____

Comments:

Evaluator's Signature: _____
Date: _____

Procedure 20-5.   Assisting Mother to Breast-Feed

Name: _____

	S	UN
1. Washed hands.	___	___
2. Had mother wash hands. Nipples were washed with plain water (if called for in care plan) in a circular motion from nipple outward.	___	___
3. Helped the mother to a comfortable position.	___	___
a. in chair with feet up on a stool	___	___
b. in bed with pillows behind back and head for support; adjusted pillows until mother was comfortable	___	___
4. Changed baby's diaper, if needed.	___	___
5. Brought baby to mother.	___	___
6. Had mother touch infant's cheek on side nearest the breast.	___	___
7. Observed that mother held back breast tissue so the baby could "latch on" to the entire nipple and most of the areola. The infant's lips covered this area. Baby's tongue was under the nipple.	___	___
8. Observed that baby nursed for about 10 minutes on each breast. If baby fell asleep during feeding, mother removed baby from breast. Awakened baby by washing face, changing diaper, or tapping feet. Put baby back to breast.	___	___
9. Reminded mother how to remove baby from breast: by inserting her finger into the corner of the baby's mouth to break the suction.	___	___
10. Observed that mother burped the baby before moving to the other breast.	___	___
11. When feeding was over, changed diaper.	___	___
12. Placed baby on right side or back.	___	___
13. Observed that mother massaged a little milk/colostrum on nipples after feeding, if desired. Breasts were air dried. Nipples were kept dry.	___	___
14. Assisted mother with dressing, if necessary. A nursing bra was worn, if desired.	___	___
15. Recorded what was done. Reported any abnormal findings to supervisor.	___	___

Comments:

Evaluator's Signature: _____
Date: _____

Procedure 20-6.   Sterilizing Bottles

Name: _____

	S	UN

1. Washed hands.
2. Obtained necessary materials.
3. Washed all bottles and nipples in dishwashing liquid and hot water. Rinsed thoroughly.
4. Placed bottles and jar of nipples in large pot. Put 2 inches (5 cm) of water in the pot. Placed lid on pot and boiled for 5 minutes. Did not lift lid during this process.
5. Let pot cool. Removed contents with tongs.
6. Stood bottles on a clean dish towel to dry.

Comments:

Evaluator's Signature: _____
Date: _____

Procedure 20-7. Preparing Formula From Powder

Name: _____

	S	UN
1. Washed hands.	___	___
2. Obtained necessary materials.	___	___
3. Boiled water and allowed to cool.	___	___
4. Poured cooled water into bottle.	___	___
5. Added powdered formula using scoop, according to label instructions.	___	___
6. Shook well to mix.	___	___
7. Capped, sealed, and stored bottles in the refrigerator until needed.	___	___

Comments:

Evaluator's Signature: _____
Date: _____

Procedure 20-8.   Preparing Formula Using Concentrated Formula

Name: _____

	S	UN
1. Washed hands.	____	____
2. Obtained necessary materials.	____	____
3. Boiled water and allowed to cool.	____	____
4. Washed can lid with hot soapy water. Rinsed. Opened can.	____	____
5. Poured appropriate amount of water into bottle.	____	____
6. Added appropriate amount of formula through funnel into bottle.	____	____
7. Shook well to mix.	____	____
8. Capped, sealed, and stored bottles in the refrigerator until needed.	____	____

Comments:

Evaluator's Signature: _____

Date: _____

Procedure 20-9.   Preparing Formula From Ready-to-Use Supply

Name: _____

	S	UN
1. Washed hands.	___	___
2. Obtained necessary materials.	___	___
3. Washed off can lid with hot soapy water. Rinsed. Opened can.	___	___
4. Poured formula into bottle using funnel.	___	___
5. Capped, sealed, and stored formula in refrigerator until needed.	___	___

Comments:

Evaluator's Signature: _____

Date: _____

Procedure 20-10. Assisting Mother to Bottle-Feed

Name: _____

	S	UN
1. Washed hands.	___	___
2. Obtained necessary materials.	___	___
3. Warmed bottle (if cold) by placing in a pan of warm water until it was about room temperature.	___	___
4. Had mother wash her hands.	___	___
5. Helped the mother to a comfortable position.	___	___
6. Changed baby's diaper, if necessary.	___	___
7. Brought bottle and baby to mother.	___	___
8. Bottle was tilted so that neck of the bottle and nipple were always covered with formula. Did not prop the bottle.	___	___
9. Had mother burp the baby halfway during the feeding and at the end.	___	___
10. Feeding was discontinued when baby was no longer eating.	___	___
11. Changed diaper.	___	___
12. Placed baby on right side or back.	___	___
13. Washed hands.	___	___
14. Recorded what was done and the amount of formula taken. Reported any unusual observations to supervisor.	___	___

Comments:

Evaluator's Signature: _____

Date: _____

Procedure 22-1.   Assisting Postoperative Client to Deep Breathe and Cough

Name: _____

	S	UN
DEEP BREATHING		
1. Explained procedure to client.		
2. Provided privacy	____	____
3. Assisted client into sitting position.	____	____
4. Had client place hands over lower end of rib cage with tips of third fingers just touching each other.	____	____
5. Instructed client to deep breathe by:	____	____
a. Exhaling until the ribs move down as far as possible.	____	____
b. Breathing in through the nose as deeply as possible. (Client should be able to feel fingers separate during inhalation.)	____	____
c. Holding the breath for a count of three.	____	____
d. Exhaling slowly through pursed lips until the ribs move as far down as possible.	____	____
6. Repeated according to care plan, usually every 1 to 2 hours while client was awake.	____	____
7. Recorded what was done. Reported any abnormal observations to supervisor.	____	____
COUGHING		
1. Explained procedure to client.	____	____
2. Asked client to place interlaced fingers or a small pillow over the incision.	____	____
3. Had client take two deep breaths.	____	____
4. Told client to take another deep breath, hold for a count of three, and then cough twice with the mouth open. Did not let client cough on aide.	____	____
5. Repeated according to care plan, usually two or three coughs per hour.	____	____
6. Recorded what was done. Reported any abnormal observations to supervisor.	____	____

Comments:

Evaluator's Signature: _____
Date: _____

Skills Competency Checklists Record

Name: _____

PROCEDURE		DATE TAUGHT	DATE SUCCESSFULLY DEMONSTRATED
10-1	Feeding the Client	____	____
11-1	Handwashing	____	____
11-2	Applying Gloves and Removing Contaminated Gloves	____	____
11-3	Disinfecting Using Wet Heat	____	____
11-4	Disinfecting Using Dry Heat	____	____
11-5	Making Bleach Solution	____	____
11-6	Making Vinegar Solution	____	____
11-7	Disinfecting With Household Solutions	____	____
11-8	Applying a Mask and Removing a Contaminated Mask	____	____
11-9	Applying a Gown and Removing a Contaminated Gown	____	____
11-10	Double Bagging	____	____
12-1	Raising Client's Head and Shoulders	____	____
12-2	Moving Client to Side of Bed	____	____
12-3	Moving Up in Bed When Client Can Help	____	____
12-4	Moving Up in Bed When Client Cannot Help	____	____
12-5	Positioning Client in Supine (Back-lying) Position	____	____
12-6	Positioning Client in Fowler's (Semi-sitting) Position	____	____
12-7	Positioning Client in Lateral (Side-lying) Position	____	____
12-8	Positioning Client in Sims' Position	____	____
12-9	Positioning Client in Prone (Abdominal) Position	____	____
12-10	Assisting Client to Sit on Side of Bed	____	____
12-11	Transferring Client From Bed to Chair/Wheelchair— Standing Transfer	____	____
12-12	Transferring Client From Bed to Chair/Wheelchair— Standing Transfer Using Transfer Belt	____	____
12-13	Returning Client to Bed	____	____
12-14	Applying a Transfer (Gait) Belt	____	____
12-15	Using a Mechanical Lift	____	____
13-1	Making a Closed Bed	____	____

PROCEDURE	DATE TAUGHT	DATE SUCCESSFULLY DEMONSTRATED
13-2 Making an Open Bed	_____	_____
13-3 Making an Occupied Bed	_____	_____
13-4 Making a Mitered Corner	_____	_____
14-1 Brushing Teeth	_____	_____
14-2 Flossing Teeth	_____	_____
14-3 Mouth Care for the Unconscious Client	_____	_____
14-4 Caring for Dentures	_____	_____
14-5 Giving a Complete Bed Bath	_____	_____
14-6 Giving a Tub Bath	_____	_____
14-7 Giving a Back Rub	_____	_____
14-8 Giving Perineal Care	_____	_____
14-9 Caring for Nails and Feet	_____	_____
14-10 Assisting Client With Hair Care	_____	_____
14-11 Giving a Shampoo	_____	_____
14-12 Shaving the Male Client	_____	_____
14-13 Helping the Client to Dress	_____	_____
14-14 Helping Client With an IV to Remove Used Clothing and Apply Clean Clothing	_____	_____
14-15 Helping With Range of Motion Exercises in Bed— General Procedure	_____	_____
15-1 Giving and Removing a Bedpan	_____	_____
15-2 Giving and Removing a Urinal	_____	_____
15-3 Measuring and Recording Intake & Output	_____	_____
15-4 Care of the Client With an Indwelling Catheter	_____	_____
15-5 Emptying a Catheter Drainage Bag	_____	_____
15-6 Applying a Condom Catheter	_____	_____
16-1 Collecting a Routine Urine Specimen	_____	_____
16-2 Collecting a "Clean Catch" Urine Specimen	_____	_____
16-3 Collecting a 24-Hour Urine Specimen	_____	_____
16-4 Straining Urine	_____	_____
16-5 Collecting a Stool Specimen	_____	_____
16-6 Collecting a Sputum Specimen	_____	_____
17-1 Cleaning a Thermometer (Glass or Oral Electronic)	_____	_____
17-2 Taking an Oral Temperature (With Glass Thermometer)	_____	_____
17-3 Taking an Oral Temperature (With Electronic Thermometer)	_____	_____
17-4 Taking an Oral Temperature (With a Single-Use Thermometer)	_____	_____

PROCEDURE	DATE TAUGHT	DATE SUCCESSFULLY DEMONSTRATED
17-5 Taking an Axillary Temperature	_____	_____
17-6 Taking a Temperature (With Tympanic Thermometer)	_____	_____
17-7 Taking a Rectal Temperature	_____	_____
17-8 Taking a Radial Pulse	_____	_____
17-9 Taking Respirations	_____	_____
17-10 Measuring Blood Pressure	_____	_____
18-1 Assisting With Oral Medications	_____	_____
18-2 Assisting With Rectal Suppositories	_____	_____
18-3 Assisting With Eye Medications or Ointment	_____	_____
18-4 Assisting With Transdermal Disks	_____	_____
18-5 Assisting With Metered-Dose Inhalers	_____	_____
18-6 Applying a Hot Water Bag	_____	_____
18-7 Applying a Hot/Cold Pack	_____	_____
18-8 Applying Hot Compresses	_____	_____
18-9 Applying Hot Soaks	_____	_____
18-10 Giving a Sitz Bath	_____	_____
18-11 Applying an Ice Bag	_____	_____
18-12 Applying Cold Compresses	_____	_____
18-13 Removing a Soiled Dressing and Applying a Clean, Dry Dressing	_____	_____
18-14 Applying Elastic Stockings	_____	_____
18-15 Applying Elastic Bandages	_____	_____
20-1 Bathing an Infant—Sponge Bath	_____	_____
20-2 Bathing an Infant—Tub Bath	_____	_____
20-3 Dressing an Infant	_____	_____
20-4 Changing a Diaper	_____	_____
20-5 Assisting a Mother to Breast-Feed	_____	_____
20-6 Sterilizing Bottles	_____	_____
20-7 Preparing Formula from Powder	_____	_____
20-8 Preparing Formula Using Concentrated Formula	_____	_____
20-9 Preparing Formula from Ready-to-Use Supply	_____	_____
20-10 Assisting Mother to Bottle-Feed	_____	_____
22-1 Assisting Postoperative Client to Deep Breathe and Cough	_____	_____

Instructor's Name:_____